QUALITATIVE RESEARCH ON SPORT AND PHYSICAL CULTURE

RESEARCH IN THE SOCIOLOGY OF SPORT

Series Editor: Kevin Young

Recent Volumes:

RESEARCH IN THE SOCIOLOGY OF SPORT   VOLUME 6

QUALITATIVE RESEARCH ON SPORT AND PHYSICAL CULTURE

EDITED BY

KEVIN YOUNG

Department of Sociology, University of Calgary, Canada

MICHAEL ATKINSON

Faculty of Physical Education and Health, University of Toronto, Canada

Emerald

United Kingdom – North America – Japan
India – Malaysia – China

Emerald Group Publishing Limited
Howard House, Wagon Lane, Bingley BD16 1WA, UK

First edition 2012

British Library Cataloguing in Publication Data
A catalogue record for this book is available from the British Library

ISBN: 978-1-78052-296-8
ISSN: 1476-2854 (Series)

ISOQAR certified
Management Systems,
awarded to Emerald for
adherence to Quality
and Environmental
standards ISO 9001:2008
and 14001:2004,
respectively

Certificate Number 1985
ISO 9001
ISO 14001

INVESTOR IN PEOPLE

CONTENTS

LIST OF CONTRIBUTORS

Carly Adams	Department of Kinesiology and Physical Education, University of Lethbridge, Lethbridge, AB, Canada
Jacquelyn Allen-Collinson	Department of Education, University of Bath, Bath, UK
Michael Atkinson	Faculty of Kinesiology and Physical Education, University of Toronto, Toronto, ON, Canada
Caroline Fusco	Faculty of Kinesiology and Physical Education, University of Toronto, Toronto, ON, Canada
Kass Gibson	Faculty of Kinesiology and Physical Education, University of Toronto, Toronto, ON, Canada
Brad Millington	Faculty of Kinesiology and Physical Education, University of Toronto, Toronto, ON, Canada
Kerrie O'Connell	Independent Artist
Emma Rich	Department of Education, University of Bath, Bath, UK
Brett Smith	School of Sport, Exercise and Health Sciences, Loughborough University, Loughborough, UK
Andrew C. Sparkes	Faculty of Education, Community and Leisure, Liverpool John Moores University, Liverpool, UK
John Sugden	School of Sport and Service Management, University of Brighton, Brighton, UK
Holly Thorpe	Faculty of Education, University of Waikato, Waikato, New Zealand

Brian Wilson   School of Kinesiology, University of British
                        Columbia, Vancouver, BC, Canada

Kevin Young   Department of Sociology, University of
                        Calgary, Calgary, AB, Canada

INTRODUCTION: THE PRACTICE OF QUALITATIVE RESEARCH AND THINKING QUALITATIVELY

Kevin Young and Michael Atkinson

Originally used simply to refer to those techniques producing 'data that are not in numerical form' (Theodorson & Theodorson, 1969, p. 326), qualitative methods expanded massively over the course of the 20th century in variety, sophistication and potential. Today, and several 'moments' (some 'blurred', others 'revolutionary' and turbulent – Denzin & Lincoln, 1994) into an already impressive history, *qualitative research* has become a broad and compelling, and yet not always easy to define, umbrella term used to refer to a constellation of descriptive and interpretive approaches. Qualitative research is, however, unambiguously 'a field of inquiry in its own right' (Denzin & Lincoln, 1994, p. 1). Their names may rarely be mentioned these days, and (sadly) contemporary 'methods' students may never study their work in the original, but qualitative methods derive from the path-breaking ventures of the early and much lauded anthropologists such as Evans-Pritchard, Radcliffe-Brown and Malinowski, as well as from the slightly later but equally path-breaking work of the mid-20th century symbolic interactionists, no one more seminal than Erving Goffman (1959, 1961, 1963).

Just as quantitative research can be pursued from varied angles, the same can be said of qualitative research. As Alasuutari (1995, p. 3) observes:

> It does not always have to mean either the traditional fieldwork based on ethnographic participant observation or in-depth interviews of a relatively small number of individuals. Interviewing techniques should be thought of much more in connection with the particular case in mind, and the degree of structure in the interviews can vary according to the particular needs. Material can also be produced in innumerable other ways ... such as [through the examination of] newspaper articles, books, advertisements and movies ... . Whatever is chosen as data, they can of course be analyzed in numerous ways.

In this way, contemporary qualitative methods eclipse the orthodoxies of interviewing and observation to include, for example documentary analysis, media analysis, visual methods, embodied methods, auto-ethnographic methods as well as triangulating within each of these approaches in the pursuit of 'mixed methods' (indeed, Denzin & Lincoln refer to qualitative methods as 'an inherently multimethod approach' – 1994, p. 2).

Taken cumulatively, qualitative methods go both broad and deep, and represent exciting potential for understanding social life. But, despite this breadth and depth, qualitative research is not, as Hesse-Biber and Leavy (2011) caution, something that can simply be learned through written explanation alone. To become a competent qualitative researcher, one has to *do it* – to train in it, to practise it directly and, needless to say, to make mistakes while doing it. As we constantly remind our students, and as one small example, if qualitative methods are practised seriously and reflected upon critically (England, 1994), the sense of anxiety and intimidation neophyte researchers take into, for instance, a first interview will evolve into an entirely more confident, fluid and better data-producing experience by the time of the 5th and 15th interview. The same applies to all methods, of course, but especially to qualitative methods where manoeuvring into the trenches of social life, however clumsily, is often tricky. The key, as the saying goes, is to get one's hands dirty, and never lose track of one's *positionality* once 'in the trenches' relative to one's respondents and research setting (England, 1994).

BRIDGING THREE 'OLOGIES'

In assembling a research design using qualitative methods, what we are really doing is building bridges between the ways that we see the world and the ways that we think it would be best examined and explained. Another way of saying this is that qualitative methods link ontology, epistemology and the Millsian sociological imagination (Mills, 1959).

Critical qualitative research tends to be guided by standard ontological assumptions about the nature of the phenomena that one wishes to investigate that have long characterised 'social definitions' paradigms (Ritzer, 1983) such as symbolic interactionism: 'reality' is created through human interaction and the ways that individuals exchange symbols; 'reality' is an outgrowth of our perceptions and the meanings we create using symbols: and, social life is comprised of multiple realties that mean different things to different people (Denzin & Lincoln, 1994). Similarly, the epistemological approach of qualitative researchers (where the relationship between evidence and knowledge is considered) is to take seriously the narratives that individuals generate as well as to understand the relationship between the researcher and respondent as a reciprocal one in which both parties are involved in a process of the *co-creation of meaning* (Denzin & Lincoln, 1994; Gubrium & Holstein, 1997). Qualitative methods are particularly well-suited for examining how social life is assigned *meaning* by individuals and groups (Hesse-Biber & Leavy, 2011). Indeed, undertaking exploratory work on social worlds where the emphasis is placed on respecting insider 'definitions of the situation' expressed using insider vocabularies is one of the principal strengths of the qualitative craft (Denzin & Lincoln, 1994). And finally, a humanistic research design requires what C. Wright Mills (1959) called a 'sociological imagination' – that is, a design that allows us to connect the social, personal and historical dimensions of people's lives. This is very difficult to do using statistics alone.

THINKING UNQUANTITATIVELY USING INTERPRETIVE TRADITIONS

It seems critical to stress two cornerstone elements of all *balanced* methodological thinking: first, quantitative and qualitative methods are not mutually exclusive and can be used in concert with one another; second, research methods should always be selected *as appropriate*. Simply stated, whether the focus is on developmental factors, mechanical factors, comparative factors or causal or predictive factors, almost any 'intellectual puzzle' can be studied using either approach (Denzin & Lincoln, 1994). While we clearly prefer thinking qualitatively and, as with most qualitative researchers, do not accept at face value massively complicated social processes, structures or experiences being reduced to a statistical probability, a mathematical score, or a table filled with dizzying correlations and associations, we respect quantitative approaches and believe that they are required to study and understand certain aspects of society, and to represent them, although admittedly in a particular kind of *reduced* way. It is certainly the case that while they occasionally overlap (as may be seen, for example, in some versions of semiotic, content, archival or phonemic analysis – Denzin & Lincoln, 1994, p. 3), quantitative and qualitative research are based on different principles and ways of *thinking* and *seeing*.

   Scholars have not always characterised the panorama of approaches
available to study society in the same way. For example, while Ritzer (1983,
pp. 434–435), borrowing from philosopher of science Thomas Kuhn (1962),
identifies three main paradigmatic approaches (one macro – the 'social facts'
paradigm, one micro – the 'social definitions' paradigm, and one behavioural
– the 'social behaviour' paradigm), Dawe (1970) speaks of 'two sociologies' –
one favouring a 'structure' approach and another favouring an 'action'
approach. These are essentially misleading divisions that have been critiqued
by theoretical sociologists aspiring to respect all 'ways of seeing' (among
others, Elias's (1987) notion of 'the hinge' stands out) in the pursuit of the
'fullest' understanding of social life. What makes Elias's 'rounded' approach
to the study of bodies in cultures distinct from many others' in the pantheon
of sociology is neither its emphasis on the historically contextual nor socially
constructed body, but rather its coupling of the culturally contoured and
intextuated body with the so-called 'natural' body (1987). Elias lobbied for a
multi-methodological and interdisciplinary programme of inquiry and
stream of theory that envisions how the physical body and its potentialities
are interwoven into social history and cultures (and indeed, vice versa) in
learned, unlearned and predominantly unplanned ways. Still, insofar as it
is useful to separate the social from the emotional and the physical, the
respective overviews of Kuhn, Dawe and others nevertheless *roughly*
outline the essential differences between the various approaches to examining
human behaviour.
   The relationship, then, between quantitative and qualitative methods and,
by extension, the relationship between their respective proponents, has
occasionally been fractious and knee-deep in stereotypes. Anyone who has
taught in a department of sociology will attest to the respective 'hierarchies
of credibility' that operate locally, and perhaps lead to office tensions
(e.g. which 'methods' courses should be privileged over others, and what
'knowledge' undergraduate and graduate students should be required to
have). Among other forms of resistance, positivists challenge qualitative
methods for being overly simplistic (even journalistic), and for producing
insignificant, non-generalisable and non-representative data and, of course,
for their flirtatious relationship with researcher bias. Even the most ardent
supporter of qualitative methods must acquiesce on the latter issue; *every*
qualitative researcher must check her data collection procedures and their
'yield' for possible bias. But things are more complicated than this. Not only
is there always the possibility of distorting researcher values and bias in
human research, but many theoretical approaches are actually unapologe-
tically 'biased', indeed assertively interventionist, and care less about

'rigour' in the positivist sense than they do about 'telling stories' about real human lives in a poignant and accessible way that lets, as Arthur Frank (2010) puts it, stories *breathe*. As Carey has noted, the positivist assumption that there is some objective truth 'out there' that can be mined using cold numerical forms – the view that there is such a thing as a value-free objectivist science – has led to the 'ever-present desire to maintain a distinction between hard science and soft scholarship' (1989, p. 99). The patronising language is telling, and the conspicuous silence around the potential biases and mistakes that can be made using *quantitative* approaches screams loudly.

Qualitative methods display and, in our view, should boast, obvious strengths. They help us understand and explain human *meanings*, and the dimensions of social life and the parts of people's lives that a Chi Square, regression analysis or a remote inferential measure cannot. As Denzin and Lincoln (1994), Berg and Lune (2012) and hoards of other methodologists have argued, *all* methods are open to distortion and malpractice, but the sorts of first-hand accounts of the social world produced by carefully executed qualitative research represent the essence of humanistic inquiry whose principal emphasis sits squarely at the door of *interpretation* and *meaning* (or hermeneutics). Reducing social life to an aggregate mathematical number where poignant fine detail and thick description (Geertz, 1973) – the Holy Grail of the interpretivist/hermeneutic tradition – get lost is simply anathema to qualitative work. The inability to delve deeply and directly into structures of meaning – how actors make sense out of their experiences and relationships – is where quantitative research struggles and qualitative research takes off.

Perhaps no one has captured the potential complexities of social life more perceptively than the great Canadian symbolic interactionist, Erving Goffman (cf. 1959, 1961, 1963). In suggesting that all human action, in any culture and any community, is constituted of both 'front' and 'back' regions, Goffman was, and is, exactly right. Whether research is designed inductively or deductively, unlike their numerical counterparts, qualitative methods provide us with the tools both for excavating in these regions as well as interpreting what goes on inside them, articulated and expressed from an insider's point of view. Sociologists and social scientists fascinated with the behind-the-scenes layers and processes of social life simply *need* qualitative methods. The search for what Weber (1949) called *verstehen* (or sympathetic understanding) is critical and inescapable. The search for verstehen in 11 different social settings, using 11 different qualitative approaches, underpins this book.

USING QUALITATIVE RESEARCH TO STUDY SPORT AND PHYSICAL CULTURE: A MEASURE OF FIT

The study of sport and physical culture, or what has sometimes been referred to as *physical cultural studies* (PCS) (Silk & Andrews, 2011) is a trans-disciplinary and multi-epistemological approach to the analysis of human movement, embodiment and corporeal representation. This encapsulates both mainstream and alternative body/sport/play/leisure cultures using a vast array of methodologies, most of them qualitative. PCS research occurs within and across cultural institutions and groups. It has emerged out of, seeks to complement, and in some ways goes beyond, long-standing sub-disciplines like the sociology of sport. PCS is theoretically driven, empirically grounded and sensitive to the prospects of working with diverse people to improve the social organisation, cultural prominence, impact and collective experience of sport, exercise, play and physical activity and education in the round. Among the many thrusts of PCS research is an emphasis on the need to study the complex sport–pleasure–body–play linkages in diverse cultural settings via an assortment of qualitative methodologies. PCS researchers often strive to produce local, national and cross-national analyses of how sport, exercise and physical activity may be contexts where social inclusion, health, safety, and human rights promotion is evident and physical, intellectual, emotional and artistic potentials are supported without fear or prejudice (Atkinson, 2011). Another way of saying this is that, via the use of qualitative methods, PCS centrally includes the study of power and social stratification. Interestingly, this is a sub-area within mainstream sociology that has historically displayed a quantitative hegemony. But this trend is changing.

With the mushrooming in many Western countries of academic programs in the sociology of sport, physical activity, exercise science, kinesiology and health, courses in research methods have expanded and diversified considerably. In many universities, methods courses at the undergraduate level must cater to students with wide ranging sub-disciplinary interests such as sociology, psychology, physiology, biomechanics, pedagogy, heath, management and others. Within this context of diversity, one of the primary pedagogical hurdles an instructor must negotiate is finding comprehensive sources on critical/qualitative methodologies in a market that contains a relative dearth of accessible and down-to-earth options. As sociology of sport, leisure and exercise studies are emerging in the United Kingdom, North America and elsewhere as an area of interest for undergraduate and graduate students, more student-friendly and innovative sources explaining qualitative methods are needed. In teaching sociology of sport and physical culture (SPC), what instructors are forced to do at present is draw from qualitative analysis chapters in commonly used sociology/sport and exercise sciences textbooks, or employ qualitative methods books from other disciplines that are simply not written for sociology of sport/sport/exercise/ health students. In our experience (we have both taught 'methods' classes for a long time (20 + and 10 + years respectively), many of these chapters/ books are neither engaging nor student-friendly, have a traditional positivistic tone and bias, and fail to clearly articulate the significance and practice of qualitative/critical methods in plain and convincing language.

What is needed, then, is a volume that outlines the main/contemporary/ cutting-edge approaches in qualitative research methods that students in undergraduate programs in sociology, sociology of sport (as well as, for instance, sport, exercise, kinesiology or health) can understand clearly. Students tend to better understand methods through the discussion of interesting, compelling or socially relevant substantive issues. Indeed, there is considerable opportunity to address classic issues in methodology, contemporary issues in research methods and innovative trends in qualitative research through case study examples from emerging and exciting areas of research in sport and physical cultural studies.

ABOUT THIS VOLUME

To this end, chapters in this volume revolve around one principal method in qualitative research, and are written in a familiar, usually first-person style. Each contributor has been asked to use her/his own substantive research to 'work through' the use of a specific method explaining, for instance, why certain methodological choices were made, what problems were faced and how these were overcome. Once again, this kind of collection, still largely absent in the sociology of sport and physical cultural studies literatures, bears real potential for use in both mainstream sociology classes as well methods classes, sociology of sport classes and other courses offered throughout the disciplines that deal with the study of sport, human movement and physical culture.

Essentially providing an overview of the field, and underscoring Rossman and Rallis' point that 'qualitative inquiry is both a science and an art' (2012, p. xv), the chapters that follow represent a comprehensive, but not exhaustive, review of qualitative research in action. They include not only conventional approaches such as ethnography, interviewing and historical and mixed methods, but also some newer perspectives that go beyond the orthodoxy of the genre such as auto-ethnography, feminist/queer methods, narrative and embodied methods, and visual methods. It is also true that in each of these methodological sub-genres there have been internal changes and impressive advances over the years, and what every one of them have to offer today is far more sophisticated in rigour and rich in potential than was previously the case. In an increasingly sensitive research climate, and a progressively transparent academy insisting on ever-more robust standards of due diligence, it is concomitantly important to consider the changing role of consent, risk and other dimensions of researcher responsibility (such as the accessing, storing and disposal of data) balanced against the realities of an often tough-to-probe community where some individuals and groups have something to hide. These factors are also considered in the respective contributions.

The chapters in this volume represent the sheer breadth and diversity of substantive research in SPC studies, and the full lexicon of qualitative methods employed in these pursuits. In Chapter 1, Carly Adams draws upon a case study of women's industrial sport in Canada to unpack the enduring significance of historical research. In the chapter, Adams makes a case for a (sociologically 'classic') method that is unnecessarily falling out of favour with contemporary sociologists of SPC. In Chapter 2, Michael Atkinson presents a similar case for combating the contemporary 'methodological amnesia' (that is, the current trend of neglecting traditional qualitative methods), in his discussion of realist ethnography. In his chapter, Atkinson discusses ethnographic methods in general, and then applies insights about performing realist ethnography on Ashtanga yoga culture in Canada. In Chapter 3, Holly Thorpe's analysis of traditional and contemporary forms of interviewing, perhaps the staple method in SPC research to date, rounds out the discussion of 'traditional' qualitative methods and provides a link to more contemporary approaches. Thorpe discusses a range of interview techniques employed with snowboarders as tools for revising extant theory on alternative/edge sports.

In Chapter 4, Smith and Sparkes introduce readers to the methodological descendant of interviewing techniques, narrative analysis. Three types of narrative analysis – holistic-content, holistic-form, and meta-auto-ethno-graphy – are the focus in their chapter. The chapter also attends to the benefits of using multiple forms of analysis and representation in narrative analysis. Rich and O'Connell's analysis of *avant garde* visual methods in

Chapter 5 discusses not only staple modes of visual analysis in recent SPC work (such as photo-voice and photo-elicitation), it also demonstrates how some are utilising visual methods to reach audiences beyond the academy. Here, the authors showcase how academic research on young people's experiences with physical education instruction itself may be integrated with arts-based modes of representation to produce socially accessible forms of knowledge. In Chapter 6, Millington and Wilson provide a case study of how young boys decode media texts about masculinities and 'interpretively' use them in order to make sense of their physical education experiences. Here, the authors illustrate the importance of media research in SPC studies, and showcase a much under-used technique in this tradition – audience ethnographic techniques.

Caroline Fusco's dissection of queer methodological epistemology and ontology in Chapter 7 showcases how SPC research can evolve as a simultaneous empirical/theoretical venture, and as an act of social intervention. This chapter discusses how 'queering' qualitative methods allows for the deconstruction of social spaces such as the locker room, and the potential destabilisation of heteronormative codes within it. An 'embodied' methodological focus is outlined in Chapter 8 by Sparkes and Smith to represent the limitations of traditional forms of inquiry and representational genres for both seeking the senses and communicating these to a range of different audiences. Here, the authors tap 'unacknowledged methodological potentialities' for probing the senses using standard methodologies, and how these might be developed further, in creative combination with more novel approaches, as part of a future shift towards more sensuous forms of scholarship in SPC. Allen-Collinson's discussion of an auto-ethnographic methodology in Chapter 9 reflects the author's seasoned experience with the technique. Building on Allen-Collinson's work on personal recovery from running injuries, the chapter provides perhaps the most detailed, reflexive and methodologically instructive analyses of the technique in the SPC literature to date.

The final two chapters of the book attend to matters often 'glossed over' or discussed mechanically or tokenistically in methods volumes. Chapter 10's discussion of mixed methodological approaches by Kass Gibson draws on the author's research on recreational athlete's relationships with performance footwear. The chapter articulates the epistemological issues and hurdles tackled in mixed methods approaches, while arguing strongly for the necessity of 'mixing methods' in many qualitative endeavours. The analysis of research ethics, investigative sociology and the search for empirical 'truths' are the foci of John Sugden's Chapter 11. Here, Sugden reflects upon a range of precarious and ethically 'complicated' field research efforts he has undertaken, in order to outline how the pursuit of empirical realities (and related sociological truth-claims) in the 'pubic interest' must be remembered as a critical mandate of the sociology of SPC.

Separately and collectively, where qualitative methods are concerned, the chapters in this volume represent an aggregate journey from conceptualisation to operationalisation. In addition to identifying the core component characteristics of each qualitative approach, they also share in common the provision of practical instructions with respect to how these methods might be implemented in the empirical setting, what problems might arise, and how they might be overcome in the pursuit of professional and sociologically-revealing interpretive practice. It is our hope that in considering these approaches, readers might find inspiration with respect to where such approaches might lead, or how to overcome complications in getting there, or simply discover new methodological angles as they take on the often inaccessible and tough-to-tackle coalfaces of social life.

REFERENCES

Alasuutari, P. (1995). *Researching culture: Qualitative method and cultural studies.* London: Sage.

Atkinson, M. (2011). Physical cultural studies (redux). *Sociology of Sport Journal, 28*, 135–141.

Berg, B. L., & Lune, H. (2012). *Qualitative research methods for the social sciences* (8th ed.). New York, NY: Pearson.

Carey, J. W. (1989). *Communication as culture: Essays on media and society.* Boston, MA: Unwin Hyman.

Dawe, A. (1970). The two sociologies. *British Journal of Sociology, 21*, 207–218.

Denzin, N. K., & Lincoln, Y. S. (1994). Introduction: Entering the field of qualitative research. In N.K. Denzin & Y.S. Lincoln (Eds.), *Handbook of qualitative research* (pp. 1–17). Thousand Oaks, CA: Sage.

Elias, N. (1987). On human beings and their emotions: A process-sociological essay. *Theory, Culture and Society, 4*, 339–361.

England, K. (1994). Getting personal: Reflexivity, positionality, and feminist research. *The Professional Geographer, 46*(1), 80–89.

Frank, A. W. (2010). *Letting stories breathe.* Chicago, IL: The University of Chicago Press.

Geertz, C. (1973). *The interpretation of cultures: Selected essays.* New York, NY: Basic Books.

Goffman, E. (1959). *The presentation of self in everyday life.* Garden City, NY: Anchor Books.

Goffman, E. (1963). *Behavior in public places.* Glencoe, IL: Free Press.

Goffman, E. (1961). *Asylums.* Garden City, NY: Anchor Books.

Gubrium, J., & Holstein, J. (1997). *The new language of qualitative method.* New York, NY: Oxford University Press.

Hesse-Biber, S., & Leavy, P. (2011). *The practice of qualitative research.* Thousand Oaks, CA: Sage.

Kuhn, T. (1962). *The structure of scientific revolutions.* Chicago, IL: University of Chicago Press.

Mills, C. Wright. (1959). *The sociological imagination.* New York, NY: Oxford University Press.

Ritzer, G. (1983). *Sociological theory.* New York, NY: Alfred A. Knopf.

Rossman, G. B., & Rallis, S. F. (2012). *Learning in the field: An introduction to qualitative research.* Thousand Oaks, CA: Sage.

Silk, M., & Andrews, D. (2011). Toward a physical cultural studies. *Sociology of Sport Journal, 28,* 4–35.

Theodorson, G. A., & Theodorson, A. G. (1969). *A modern dictionary of sociology.* New York, NY: Thomas Cromwell Company.

Weber, M. (1949). *The methodology of the social sciences.* In E. Shils & H. Finch (Eds.), New York, NY: Free Press.

CHAPTER 1

HISTORICAL METHODS
AND TRACES OF THE PAST:
EMBRACING THE COMPLEXITIES
AND ENGAGING IN
REFLEXIVITY

Carly Adams

ABSTRACT

Purpose – *This chapter explores various approaches to historical methods as they relate to sport and physical culture research.*

Design/methodology/approach – *The chapter discusses various paradigmatic approaches to historical methods (reconstructionist, constructionist and deconstructionist) and takes up current debates related to archives, newspapers, photographs and oral history as they relate to the method. Drawing on these discussions, I outline various approaches to designing a sport and physical culture project using historical methods, focusing on my work on women's industrial sport in the 1920s and early 1930s.*

Findings – *I discuss how data evolved from the method and how I made choices about the inclusion and exclusion of materials. The chapter*

Qualitative Research on Sport and Physical Culture
Research in the Sociology of Sport, Volume 6, 1–21
Copyright © 2012 by Emerald Group Publishing Limited
All rights of reproduction in any form reserved
ISSN: 1476-2854/doi:10.1108/S1476-2854(2012)0000006004

concludes that historical methods are tedious, complex and messy but also exciting and insightful ways to do research. I also conclude by encouraging the researcher to be reflexive and aware of one's 'positionality' as a researcher and embrace the historical process.

Originality/value – *The chapter is original work. It is not so much a prescriptive 'how-to' guide for historical research, but it works to take up current debates in historical methods. It also endeavours to engage students and scholars alike as they consider their research projects and the potential value of historical methods.*

Keywords: Historical methods; paradigms; archives; oral history; newspapers; photographs

INTRODUCTION

My first answer therefore to the question, What is history? is that it is a continuous process of interaction between the historian and [her] facts, an unending dialogue between the present and the past. E. H. Carr (1969, p. 35).

Over the last decade, there has been increasing recognition of the historical, cultural and social significance of the active body among scholars in the humanities and social sciences. Physical cultural theorist David Andrews (2008) suggests that the 'ontological complexity of physical culture ... encourages a methodological dynamism that requires the ... researcher to become proficient within a range of qualitative and interpretive approaches' (p. 57). Historical methods, as part of sport and physical culture research, are used to take up how we understand the body and physical movement as we (re/de)construct assumptions about the past. Through this method, we look at a wide array of traces[1] of the past (such as those found in archives, mass media, material culture) to examine the active body, and the ways subjective, embodied identities and experiences are negotiated in specific socio-historical contexts (Andrews, 2008; Hargreaves & Vertinsky, 2007). An understanding of historical methods is essential for students embarking on sport and physical culture research projects. The purpose of this chapter, then, is to discuss various approaches to historical methods as they relate to sport and physical culture.

PARADIGMATIC APPROACHES

All social phenomena, interactions and behaviours have histories – our understanding of the present must be contextualised and situated within an understanding of the past. Historical work begins by identifying one's approach or paradigmatic position. Nancy Struna (2010) writes that a paradigm is 'an intellectual device that contains scholarly beliefs and assumptions about the world, the past, and the evidence' (p. 203). Two questions one might consider are, for example, what are my views on theory and data collection and what research questions will I pursue? A consideration of one's ontological and epistemological assumptions guides us as we do our work. Drawing on the work of historian Alan Munslow (1997), sports historian Doug Booth (2005) suggests that in historical work examining sport and physical culture, there are three models of historical inquiry – reconstructionism, constructionism and deconstructionism. These three perspectives influence the objectives of our research, the approaches we take and how we present our findings. Reconstructionists strive to discover the truth about the past, as it 'actually happened' or 'it really was' (Booth, 2005, p. 9). Reconstructionists are intent on interrogating and checking the credibility of traces of the past to verify that they are real and true and presenting history in coherent prose narratives. From this perspective, one maintains that history exists 'independent of the researcher'. It is a process that is objective and simply a relaying of facts without any interpretation (Booth, 2005; Munslow, 1997; Stanford, 1994). Similarly, constructionists value empirical facts as the fundamental source for 'knowing' the past. As Booth (2005) suggests, 'reconstructionism and constructionism are evidence-based, objectivist-inspired models in which historians aspire to build accurate, independent and truthful reconstructions of the past' (p. 10). However, these two models diverge in that for constructionists, theoretical engagement with the past is essential in historical research. From this perspective, one's theoretical framework is a critical tool for selecting appropriate traces of the past to enhance our understandings of the past. Deconstructionists, on the other hand, do not believe in the notion of objectivity or the idea of the historian as an objective researcher (Booth, 2005; Munslow, 1997). Deconstructionists examine different views of an historical moment and stress that all historical understandings are partial, fluid and subjective (e.g. Phillips, 2002). Choices that historians make relate to how we frame our research questions, design our projects, interpret the past and present our findings have important ideological and political implications (Booth, 2005; White, 1973).

TRACES OF THE PAST

Historical work is dependent on (1) the 'traces' of the past that are available to the researcher and (2) as Peter Burke (2001) suggests, the intermediaries – other historians, archivists and witnesses, for example – who have recorded or preserved the past in particular ways. The range of traces of the past considered for a particular project will also depend on the research topic, paradigmatic approach and interests of the researcher. For each project, we need to select and identify the most appropriate traces of the past. Indeed, all historical research involves tough ontological and epistemological choices (Booth, 2005; White, 1973). Not all researchers employing historical methods approach history or their interpretation and analysis of traces of the past in the same way. As Booth (2005) explains:

> reconstructionists treat historical materials as concrete facts and interrogate them to ascertain their truthfulness; constructionists contextualise historical materials within theoretical frameworks that they hold as the primary means by which historians reveal reality; deconstructionists conceptualise historical materials as discourses and texts, and search these linguistic forms for their inherent power relations. (p. 82)

Deconstructionists argue that all traces of the past are inextricably linked to social power. Regardless of one's paradigmatic position, a researcher employing historical methods must critically consider as much as possible about the origins and content of each document or object as a trace of the past. Who wrote it? When? Why? Who was the audience?

EXPLORING THE ARCHIVES: (UN)OFFICIAL DOCUMENTS

Archives are the bread and butter of historical work. What you find at an archive may include official published documents such as government records, parliamentary debates, reports of governmental inquires or commissions, census data, magazines, newspapers, maps as well as unofficial or unpublished documents such as meeting minutes, organisational memos, memoirs, diaries, correspondence and photographs. Archives can be found in people's basements, closets, an organisation's storage room or in meticulously organised public buildings. The type of archive could range from local/regional such as private collections, historical societies, municipal collections, sports halls of fame or institutes of higher learning to public national and international archives. Sport historian Robert Barney's (1995) concise how-to guide for researchers new to the archival environment provides practical information on how to identify the appropriate archives, how to plan for the visit, considerations for working in an archive and post-visit concerns.

Digging (sometimes literally) through archival 'fonds' (collections of documents on a particular subject) is often a daunting and tedious task. But, coming face to face with traces of the past is exhilarating and rewarding (Barney, 1995). As researchers, however, we need to be aware of the gaps and omissions in archives, as archives function as spaces for both preservation and exclusion (Ballantyne, 2003; Booth, 2005; Burton, 2005; Hamilton, Harris, & Reid, 2002). Hamilton et al. (2002) argue that the archive is 'figured' and it is 'always already being refigured' (p. 7). They argue, 'the technologies of creation, preservation and use, for instance, are changing all the time; physically the archive is being added to and subtracted from, and is in dynamic relation with its physical environment; organisational dynamics are ever shifting; and the archive is porous to societal processes and discourses' (Hamilton et al., 2002, p. 7). As with all traces of the past, we must consciously engage and continually question the origin and purpose of documents and materials in archives (Booth, 2005, p. 87). How is knowledge of the past produced?

NEWSPAPERS

There are many forms of mass communication potentially used as traces of the past for historical work, including newspapers, magazines, posters and Internet sites. Unlike archival sources that are often unpublished or printed in small numbers, documents of mass communication are printed in large quantities for mass distribution in hard copy or electronically. This section will focus on the potential and problems of newspapers as traces of the past since they constitute arguably the most common form of mass communication examined by historians of sport and physical culture. Also, for students, newspapers are perhaps the traces of the past most easily and readily accessible (Booth, 2005). Newspapers often offer day-to-day coverage of events. They provide information about sporting events (dates, times, venues), results and scores, the names of players, coaches and officials. But articles, letters, editorials and photographs also offer insights into political, cultural and social thinking, conventions, and values of the time. Local and national newspapers contribute to constructing understandings of the active body during specific socio-historical periods of time.

Newspapers, although commonly accepted as important sources of information about the past, pose an array of challenges for historians. Often considered as first-hand accounts of events of the past, newspaper articles, columns and editorials are written with the intent of selling a product to an audience (Franzosi, 1987; Hill, 2006). Yet, newspapers, like other historical traces, provide, as Hill (2006, p. 119) explains, a 'point of access' to the past. Indeed, in some cases, the newspaper may constitute the only available trace of the past. Newspapers, like other forms of media, are sites of ideological power and as such, as we examine these traces of the past, we must consider newspapers as a mediated text and ask questions about the control over the production process and the possible manipulation of representations within the text (Birrell & Theberge, 1994; Booth, 2005). What is the political position of the newspaper and editors? Who wrote the article? Why? Who was its intended audience?

PHOTOGRAPHS

Some historians continue to note the reluctance of researchers to engage with the complexities of meaning that photographs represent (Burke, 2001; Cashman, 1995; Fyfe & Law, 1988; Gaskell, 1991). Traditional historical methods tend to use photographs to illustrate predetermined conclusions. In 2008, Mike Huggins questioned: 'Have the more theoretical aspects of the broader "visual turn" in cultural studies reached sport history?' (p. 313). Huggins (2008) suggests that although an engagement with the visual in sport history is sometimes 'ghettoized on the margins of the field', more and more historians of sport and physical culture are taking up and theorising the visual (e.g. Bale, 1998; Brown, 2007; Constanzo, 2002; Huggins & O'Mahony, 2011; Oriard 1993, 2001; O'Mahony, 2006; Osmond, 2008, 2010; Phillips, O'Neill, & Osmond, 2007; Schultz, 2006).

Photographs are more than merely illustrative representations of conclusions. They are not objective renderings of events as one may think upon first glance. Rather, they are constructed in specific ways, often for a specific purpose, at a specific moment in time. They are traces of the past that act as significant arbitrators of meaning (e.g. Osmond, 2008; Thyssen, 2007). Just as E. H. Carr (1969) argued that we must study the historian before we study the facts, so too must we study the purpose of a photograph. We must ask questions such as the following: Why was it taken? By whom? For what audience? While many of these questions are often left unanswered, or are in some cases unanswerable, it is important to recognise that photographs

render experiences of physical embodiment visible. They capture a particular point of view and perspective. Sport historian Gary Osmond (2008)
suggests that 'as material objects that are produced and reproduced in
various media, that are viewed in different contexts, appropriate to various
tasks, recycled and invented, photographs and their images inevitably
change' (p. 342). The content of the photograph is, of course, an important
trace of history (Burke, 2001). What is the person/group doing? What are
they wearing? Who is in the photograph and who is not? What does the
background tell us? Edwards and Hart (2004) suggest this is the most
straightforward way we think about and engage with photographs; this is
why collections of photographs are so important, why they are valued as
gifts, or preserved in scrapbooks or photo albums. However, we need to go
beyond this to consider the materiality of the photograph – the physical
aspects of the image.

Photographs often end up in scrapbooks or photo boxes and are handed
down from generation to generation, or are donated to libraries and
archives for safekeeping. As Osmond (2008) suggests, these acts of recycling
position photographs as arbitrators of meaning and provide different
meanings depending on the place, time and context. The process of creating
scrapbooks is an interesting way photographs are recycled. Scrapbooks are
individualised and personal acts of preserving photographs and news images
in particular ways. They often indicate as much about the person putting it
together as about the subject matter itself. While we may never know the
intent of the sequencing or selection of scrapbook materials, they clearly
indicate an individual's engagement with a life story (Osmond, 2008).

Let us pause for a moment and think about newspaper photographs and
the varied meanings they can impart. Newspaper photographs are clearly
textually dependent. The picture is often framed by words and particular
layouts that influence the meaning that is relayed to readers. As Osmond
(2008) suggests: 'while photographic content is obviously important to
interpretation, image alone is not the sole repository of meaning' (p. 346).
Photographic images 'cannot be fully understood at any single point in its
existence but should be understood as belonging in a continuing process of
production, exchange, usage and meaning' (Edwards & Hart, 2004, p. 4).
The meanings attached to an image when it appeared in a newspaper in the
1930s, for example, are very different from the meanings the photographs
hold for family members who recycle the images from generation to
generation, or researchers deconstructing the past. Archived materials, such
as photographs and scrapbooks, not only preserve – they reify, frame and
set meaning. Images are material objects. They are socially constructed

within the context of time and they are loaded with symbolic meaning, hidden complexities and subjective perceptions. Offering snapshots of certain moments of time, photographs often provide more questions than answers. It is the posing of new questions that challenges and expands traditional understandings of physical embodiment and identity negotiation in specific socio-historical contexts.

ORAL HISTORIES

Early works of historical scholarship rarely made use of oral histories as traces of the past. Susan Cahn (1994b) suggests that this may have been due to the structural focus of sport historians' research questions in the late 1970s and 1980s and the focus on sport in the 19th century (e.g. Guttmann, 1978; Hardy, 1982; Metcalfe, 1987; Radar, 1983). However, by the mid-1980s, there were some exceptions as scholars used oral histories (often as traces of the past among other traces of the past) to broaden understandings of sport and recreation in particular moments in time or in biographical accounts of individual athletes (e.g. Allen, 1985; Baker, 1986; Rosenzweig, 1983). By the 1990s, oral history became an important method for research into gender and women's experiences related to sport and physical culture (e.g. Cahn, 1994a; Hargreaves, 1994). Although it could be argued that most historical work continues to privilege written accounts, oral reminiscences are increasingly gaining acceptance as legitimate traces of the past. Booth (2005) suggests that those from a reconstructionist approach seek to remain detached to obtain objective facts from oral accounts, while deconstructionists locate oral accounts and reminiscences in particular cultural practices and embrace the co-constructed nature of oral interviews (Thomson, 1998).

Oral histories – the recording and analysis of oral interpretations of the past – are complex, time consuming but immensely rewarding undertakings when investigating sport and physical culture. There is no prescription or 'best practice' for this type of work. Oral narratives are unique, fluid and situated. They work to create space for absent subjects and experiences while challenging and deconstructing traditional understandings of the active body. Oral interviews constitute an important part of historical analysis, as an individual's personal narrative serves as a link between her/his personal experiences and the socio-historical time of which s/he was a part (Thompson, 2000). If we decide to conduct oral histories as part of our research projects, as researchers we are making specific analytical choices about which voices, identities and stories will be central to the research (and which ones may be silenced).

Historian Alessandro Portelli (1991) argues that 'oral sources tell us not just what people did, but what they wanted to do, what they believed they were doing, and now what they think they did' (p. 50). Geiger (1991) suggests that oral history only 'becomes a *method* in the hands of the researcher' (p. 170). Returning to my earlier discussion about paradigmatic positions in historical work related to sport and physical culture, oral histories are a feminist method based on my underlying reasons for collecting these oral histories and in the way I use them (Sangster, 1997). In my work, I adopted several theoretical and related methodological tenets: gender is an important central analytical concept; women's experiences and perspectives embody and create historically and situationally specific realities and work to deconstruct and unsettle other understandings of sport history; I recognise and advocate women's own interpretations of their experiences and social worlds as containing and reflecting important understandings of the past.[2] My assumptions influence the kinds of questions I ask and my motivations for conducting certain oral histories. I actively choose to pursue my oral history projects and the stories of the people I speak to as the *topic* of analysis not as a *resource* for my analysis (Rapley, 2004). In my work, I am committed to oral history research and the importance and potential of the co-constructed narrative.

DESIGNING A PROJECT

The most important part of any research project, and the starting point, is to determine the topic of investigation. To do this, keep in mind the required scope of the project, your objectives and your own personal interests. Once you have determined the topic (even if it is only in the broadest sense), a thorough literature search of relevant secondary sources is the next step to find out what has been researched and written about or related to the topic. Online databases such as SPORTdiscus or Sociological Abstracts allow quick searching using keywords related to your topic. Reading as much as possible that has been published related to the topic will allow you to identify what other scholars have researched and argued related to your topic and, perhaps, more importantly, gaps in the literature. By thoroughly examining the notes and references from the secondary literature, you will be able to determine relevant primary traces of the past that you may want to look at for your project. Also, from the secondary sources often comes the development of research questions that will frame and direct the project. Struna (2010) argues that a good historical research question is one that is derived from the literature. Once the questions are developed, we need to identify the evidence needed to answer them. Will you draw on official documents, diaries, newspapers? Will you conduct oral history interviews?[3]

Once you have located the traces of the past you will use and conducted and transcribed the oral history interviews (if applicable), the next step is to scrutinise the traces. What do they tell you about the research question you have identified? It is also important to put the evidence you have collected in the context of your secondary sources. How does your evidence support or refute the arguments that others have made? The next (and arguably most important) step in historical research is making sense of, or interpreting, what you found. There is no one way to do this. There are, potentially, as many ways to interpret evidence as there are historians or research projects. Your paradigmatic approach and the theoretical frameworks you will use to deconstruct and analyse the traces of the past that you have collected will drive the process of interpretation and analysis.

What I outline above is the (linear) advice most often prescribed for historical research. In practice, though, it often does not look as 'neat' as this. For example, on many occasions, I have stumbled upon research topics while digging in an archive looking for something related to another project. It is often a muddled, circuitous process that goes back and forth and not in a linear step one, then step two progression.

For the purposes of this chapter and by way of example, I discuss how I approached and designed a project examining women's industrial softball in London, ON, from 1923 to 1935 (Adams, 2011a). This project is part of a larger study that set out to examine women's sport in the city through three case studies: the municipal playground movement, industrial softball leagues and city-organised leagues, resulting in several conference presentations and three peer-reviewed publications (Adams, 2011a, 2011b, 2006). This project evolved and changed through the course of the research and writing. By using this project, and discussing the shifts in design from design to publication, I aim to highlight and speak to some of the important practical decisions we make in the course of historical research.

When I first began the project, the broad purpose of the study was to investigate the experiences of women who played sport in London, ON, from 1920 to the early 1950s in order to provide greater insight on women's social experiences through the meaning they attached to their active bodily practices. The questions that guided this study during the planning and designing stages included the following: How do women remember and relate their sport experiences of the past? What meanings did individual women draw from their sport involvement? How can we understand women's sport communities historically? How did women embrace and challenge notions of community? How did women and men react to the social challenges posed by women's athletic participation? How do oral histories, newspapers and photographs influence our perceptions of women's sport?

At the outset of this project, I encountered the pervasive practical problem of writing about women's sport experiences of the past, particularly in smaller urban and rural communities – the perceived dearth of available traces of the past. For certain topics and periods of women's sport participation in London, there was an abundance of traces. However, for other periods, very little written material was available. As a researcher dedicated to historical methods, I had to make complex and important decisions about which traces to include and what to leave out. Historical research requires that we consider the materials that are available and to interrogate and take these up in ways that, to some, may be considered as non-traditional historical analysis. Contextualised within relevant secondary sources from history, sociology and sport studies to situate women's sport within the broader social context, my objective for this project was to draw on as many traces of the past as possible while considering simultaneously not only what information was available through these traces of the past but how it was delivered and the variety of meanings embedded in each.

I would now like to turn my attention specifically to the industrial sport piece of this project by way of providing a more precise example, and to take up some of the ideas and complexities mentioned above. Emphasising the notion that all traces of the past are inextricably linked to social power, this study set out to weave together oral accounts, newspaper reports, photographic representations and available archival materials. I started by conducting a thorough literature review on working women during the 1920s and 1930s (e.g. Sangster, 1995; Strong-Boag, 1979), industrial recreation (e.g. Fones-Wolf, 1986; Gems, 2001), women's industrial sport and recreation (e.g. Emery, 1994; Forbes, 2001; Sangster, 1993) and the notion of corporate welfarism (e.g. Hunnicutt, 1996; Yacob, 2008; Zahavi, 1998). From this reading, I started to form a tentative research question: How did women negotiate their work, sport, educational and family obligations within the context of corporate welfare strategies employed by London companies in the 1920s and early 1930s? Through my reading, I also decided that women's voices needed to be central to the project. So, although other traces of the past (such as organisational documents and news reports) were important, oral histories of the women who participated were central to my analysis and to my conclusions. I sought to consider the constructions of meaning that shape our understanding of the leisure time pursuits of working women in the city and the meaning it has for them decades later.

After a comprehensive literature review, my next step was a day-by-day analysis of local London newspaper reports from *The Free Press* from 1923 to 1935. *The Free Press*, the most widely circulated newspaper in the city since the late 1800s, constituted an important source of longitudinal and often day-to-day coverage of women's industrial softball leagues during this period. News coverage was extensive, with dozens of articles, editorial commentaries and game advertisements each season promoting the teams and league opponents. As early as 1922, newspaper reports offered brief references to women's exhibition games between companies such as Woolworths and Smallman & Ingram's. By 1924, organised softball was well established in the city with two leagues and eighteen teams (Adams, 2011a).

As I spent months reading microfilmed newspaper articles, I was surprised by what I was reading in the actual coverage of the industrial leagues. From my literature review, I had become familiar with Helen Lenskyj's (1987) argument that journalists, during the interwar years, commented explicitly on appearance and offered an array of personal anecdotal information about female athletes, such as their marital status and personality traits, which suggested to the reader that sport was not stripping women of their feminine attributes. Yet, in *The Free Press* during the 1920s and into the 1930s, reporting on women's softball was for the most part devoid of these stereotypical depictions. Indeed, my analysis suggested that there was very little information about the players at all, no textual reference to their appearance, their private lives as single women or even their work positions. Indeed, if first names or feminine signifiers were not provided, one would be hard pressed to determine the sex of the athletes, as evident in the following examples:

> The heavy-hitting business college girls collected a total of 13 hits off pitcher R. Jamieson. Home Runs by Phyllis Hall and Lottie Armstrong featured the game while the latter player was the leading hitter securing a home run, a triple and a single out of four chances. ('Major Girl Loop's Standing Closer', *The Free Press* (London, ON), August 2, 1929, p. 11)

> The Thistles batters collected a total of 13 hits off Pitcher Lillian Horlick. Jean Topping made the only home run of the game in the second inning with no bases occupied; while

Verna Sumner hit for three bases in the first frame with one on base. Hazel Shackleton of Rideau Hall made a double. ('Wells Academy Defeat All Stars', *The Free Press* (London, ON), August 17, 1927, p. 10)

The Purples took the lead in the first inning, when Viola King was safe on Dorothy Gardiner's error and was sacrificed on Alexander's bunt. Sadie Watson walked and King scored on an infield out. During this no one paid attention to Sadie Watson, and she stole home for the second Purple run of the inning. ('Fifth Straight Win for the St. Thomas Girls', *The Free Press* (London, ON), August 24, 1932, p. 13)

There seemed to be different prescribed notions of appropriate femininity for the working women, predominantly from the working class, who are the subjects of this investigation, and the middle-class women who so often are the subjects of historical scholarship on women's sport. Working women in smaller urban areas, at least as evident by reporting in *The Free Press*, seemed to escape the social criticism based on their femininity or perceived lack of it that their counterparts faced in major Canadian cities.

After this extensive newspaper review, I turned my attention to oral accounts. I decided to publish an article in the reader-to-reader section of the local paper, the *London Free Press*, indicating that I was interested in speaking to women who played industrial softball in the city during the 1920s and 1930s. As a result of this advertisement, I received dozens of phone calls and letters from people living in London and the surrounding area offering photographs, scrapbooks and anecdotes of mothers, aunts, friends and sisters who competed in the industrial leagues. I was overwhelmed by the response. Through these exchanges, I was able to identify and contact Hazel Shackleton, Gladys Oliver, Olive Campbell, Bertha Bradford – four women who played on various London industrial-sponsored teams during the 1920s and 1930s. The interviews with these women were approximately two to three hours in length and were sometimes followed up with telephone calls. The interviews took place in the homes of the interviewees or in a convenient location in close proximity to the interviewees' homes. During the interviews, the women often shared scrapbooks, and other articles such as uniforms, trophies and memorabilia that could provide additional insight to their experiences.

I also decided to analyse as many photographic representations of women's industrial softball as I could find. I sought to collect these through the local archives and also personal collections that I encountered through oral history interviews. Over 300 photographs were collected from *The Free Press*, and the personal scrapbooks of the athletes who I interviewed as part of the project. The photographs were visual traces of the past. Offering snapshots of certain moments of time, photographs often provide more questions than answers. Finally, archival sources from the archives of the J. J. Talman regional collection at The University of Western Ontario, including the Public Utilities Commission records, municipal meeting minutes, company annual reports and newsletters, and photographs were also important traces of the past.

FROM DATA TO ANALYSIS

Once I collected the data, I had to make some decisions about its analysis and representation. How do I analyse and make sense of all of these traces of the past? Although some authors offer prescriptive ways for doing an analysis of historical material (e.g. Struna, 2010), in reality, this can be a messy, meandering adventure. I often start by identifying common themes across all of the material I have collected. Most often these themes relate to my initial research question(s) but sometimes they do not. For example, an interesting theme emerged in *The Free Press* during the 1920s and 1930s and in my interviewees' narratives – the acceptance and normalisation of injury and pain in women's softball of this period. It seemed that in the sporting culture of women's industrial softball in the 1920s and 1930s, serious injuries were relatively commonplace. Newspapers of the era commonly reported broken bones, lacerations, twisted knees and collisions that left players unconscious. The women I interviewed also offered similar narratives. Referring to her experiences playing softball in the late 1920s, Bertha Bradford recalled,

> I never had a glove ... I broke that finger. At the time I said to somebody, I think I have done something to that finger. Oh no, it's just sprained. So, I went around for about a week and didn't do anything about that finger. Finally I went to a doctor. He says you have broken that finger ... so he put a cast on it.

Journalists generally framed injury-related stories within the context of a fast-paced or exciting game on the diamond, naturalising injuries as an incidental part of the game. I also read reports that celebrated pain tolerance. For example, at the Western Ontario girl's softball championship in Woodstock on August 24, 1924:

> An unfortunate incident occurred in the fifth inning of this game, when Audrey McCready, the crack pitcher of the Jersey Creams had her head badly cut when she collided with Emily Poole, the catcher. She was carried off the field in an unconscious condition and, although she lost a considerable amount of blood, she recovered

sufficiently to proceed to London later in the evening. ('London Red Arrows Win Girls' Soft Ball Tourney', *The Free Press* (London, ON), August 25, 1924, p. 9)

From these stories I questioned: Were these stories fictional or embellished for entertainment value? How did these representations support or challenge understandings of femininity and more specifically athletic femininity during the 1920s and early 1930s?

Another interesting finding relating to injuries was the stories of financial compensation for pain and suffering. I first came across references in the newspaper reports. News reports in the early 1930s suggested that there was a system of insurance for injured players. For example, fundraising exhibition games were arranged in honour of injured players, with a portion of the gate receipts dedicated to hospital expenses. In May 1931, *The Free Press* reported: 'Group insurance for players will be carried by the league this year, and it is planned to play exhibition games in St. Thomas and London to assist in this fund' ('To Install New Field at Tecumseh Park', *The Free Press* (London, ON), May 6, 1931, p. 18). During a time when subsidised health care was not available, a makeshift health care insurance was offered for players who risked injury for the success of the team. This system of financial compensation was set up to compensate women for expenses incurred through hospital bills and lost wages, and suggests that practices associated with professional ideologies could perhaps be found in women's sport in the late 1920s and early 1930s. Building on this, I then asked the interviewees to speak to their personal memories of injuries and related financial support. A player for the Kellogg's team from 1928 until 1932, Gladys Oliver recalled: 'We had what they called an injured players fund ... Well, if a girl got injured her expenses and her doctor's bill and that were covered through the insurance. We were covered by insurance for that'. In the sporting subcultures of women's industrial softball, injuries were normalised and expected during the course of the season or during an intensely competitive match. Perhaps, playing through pain and injury was an important part of creating and sustaining player reputations as credible ball players. Certainly, news reports related stories of injury and financial support as part of the women's softball story. Stories about intense competition and resulting injuries were a part of the reminiscences of the women interviewed for this study.

I also examined other themes such as memories of recruitment, team loyalty, familial commitments, agency and social freedom, and representations of appropriate femininities. For the women involved in sport in London during this period, these moments of organised play were what Mona Gleason (1999) calls 'significant arbitrators of experience' (p. 113). As

I set out to make sense of these experiences (or themes, as I loosely labelled them), I began by contextualising the data and to do this I went back to my literature review. However, I had some important decisions to make. Should I focus on my original topic and research question? Should I explore new themes that I had identified and thus go back and expand my literature review? I had to make tough choices about what to leave in and what to exclude. In the end I decided to focus on my initial research question as outlined above. This meant, however, that some of the important themes and stories (such as the representations of injury and pain) were set aside for further investigation in the future.

The women's memories of playing industrial softball during this era spoke to the ways they understood their active bodies as sites of negotiation. The employers created an environment of support and financial means through providing jobs, privileges and in some cases tuition. The women in exchange felt a sense of obligation to stay with the company which hired them. To some extent, the women understood themselves as company commodities. They were bought and hired for a specific purpose – to win softball games. From this study, I concluded that, similar to Sangster's (1993) findings, at the core of the women's experiences were paternalistic practices in the guise of corporate welfarism. But their stories went beyond notions of obligation. These women were actively weighing options and figuring out what made sense for them and committing their loyalties to team or family based on their personal values and the pleasure of their active bodies.

CONCLUSION

Historical methods present many challenges and potentials to SPC researchers. Certainly it is a tedious, time-consuming endeavour to collect, critically analyse and engage with traces of the past. When using historical methods, we need to be constantly engaging in a process of questioning our assumptions and the traces we have in front of us to offer alternative perspectives and understandings of the past. Most importantly, we must remember that our interpretation is not *the* interpretation but it is merely *one* perspective on a moment in time. As researchers, we are always making choices about what to include and what not to include and how to interpret and present our work.

Growing numbers of researchers who employ historical methods are locating themselves in their work. Drawing on the work of Berkhofer (1995), Booth (2005) argues that a 'fully reflexive historian will engage with her or his ontology, epistemology, sources, theory, ethics, morality, politics, viewpoints, concept of time and space, context, narrative, rhetoric, genre and field' (p. 212). Encouraged by new work in physical cultural studies (e.g. Giardina & Newman, 2011), I suggest that when engaging in historical work we must be reflexive and aware of our positionality as researchers and embrace this as part of the research process. Historical methods are complex and often messy. This type of work involves patience and openness to engage in new ideas and understandings of particular moments and a willingness to challenge our complicity in producing and reproducing particular understandings of the past. We need to contextualise, problematise and historicise all traces of the past. Most importantly, despite the information I have offered above, I am in no way suggesting that there is a definitive way to use historical methods in sport and physical culture research. As you embark on your own project, I encourage you to embrace the exciting complexities and messiness of historical work.

FIVE KEY READINGS

1. Booth, D. (2005). *The field: Truth and fiction in sport history.* **New York: Routledge.**
Booth offers a detailed analysis of the field of sport history, exploring the questions researchers ask and the approaches and techniques used in historical methods. This book is an important source in that it details a variety of approaches to historical work, offers an extensive bibliography and speculates on the future of the field.

2. Burke, P. (2001). *Eyewitnessing: The uses of images as historical evidence.* **Ithaca, NY: Cornell University Press.**
Burke explores the use of images as historical evidence, offering a discussion on the pitfalls and potentials of material culture as traces of the past. Exploring a variety of time periods and types of images (art, photographs, advertisements, etc.), the author discusses iconography, iconology, representations of power and protest, stereotypes and the cultural history of images in an insightful study of historical method.

3. Burton, A. (2005). *Archive stories: Facts, fictions, and the writing of history.* **Durham, NC: Duke University Press.**
In this edited collection, Burton and colleagues offer engaging ethnographies of archival encounters. Through 16 provocative stories, the authors challenge us to critically analyse our archival journeys as we take up topics such as how archives are constructed, manipulated and experienced.

4. Phillips, M. G. (2006). *Deconstructing sport history: A postmodern analysis.* **Albany, NY: State University of New York Press.**
In this edited collection, Phillips and colleagues offer an insightful look at theory, practice and the future of sport history. Contributors Alun Munslow, Douglas Booth, Brett Hutchins, Michael Oriard, John Bale, Jeffery Hill, Catriona Parratt, Steven Pope, Robert Rinehart, Synthia Sydnor, Patricia Vertinsky and Murray Phillips challenge the reader to take up new approaches and challenge accepted understandings and practices in historical work.

5. Thompson, P. (2000). *The voice of the past: Oral history.* **New York: Oxford University Press.**
Thompson, one of the pre-eminent scholars in historical research and oral history method, offers an invaluable discussion on the meaning of history and situates oral history work within the broader history community. This book is the formative work for students embarking on oral history offering a theoretical engagement with the method while also providing a how-to-guide for designing the project, conducting the interviews and interpreting the narratives.

NOTES

1. Drawing on the work of Dutch historian Gustaaf Renier (see Reneir, G. (1950). *History: It's Purpose and Method.* London: Allen & UnWin), Peter Burke advocates using the phrase 'traces of the past' instead of sources. The term 'source' is problematic in that implies that there is the possibility of a 'truthful' or 'real' account of the past, which is untainted by intermediaries. The term 'trace' is more inclusive and can refer to official and unofficial documents, oral testimonies, photographs, monuments, buildings, etc.
2. This list was influenced by Susan Geiger's work (1991).
3. In the event that you decide to conduct oral interviews, you will need to seek approval from your institutional research ethics board and consent from the interview participants. See Boschma, G., Yonge, O., & Mychajlunow, L. (2003). Consent in oral history interviews: Unique challenges. *Qualitative Health Research,* 13(1), 129–135.

REFERENCES

Adams, C. (2006). Softball and the female community: Pauline Perron, pro ball player, outsider, 1926–1951. *Journal of Sport History,* *33*(3), 323–343.
Adams, C. (2011a). 'I just felt like I belonged to them': Women's industrial softball, London, Ontario, 1923–1935. *Journal of Sport History,* *38*(1), 401–417.

Adams, C. (2011b). Supervised places to play social reform, citizenship, and femininity at municipal playgrounds in London, Ontario, 1900–1942. *Ontario History, 103*(1), 60–80.

Allen, J. (1985). Values and sport: The development of New England skiing 1870–1940. *Oral History Review, 13*, 55–76.

Andrews, D. (2008). Kinesiology's inconvenient truth and the physical cultural studies imperative. *Quest, 60*, 46–63.

Baker, W. J. (1986). *Jesse Owens: An American life*. New York: University of Illinois Press.

Bale, J. (1998). Capturing 'The African' body: Visual images and 'imaginative sports'. *Journal of Sport History, 25*(2), 234–251.

Ballantyne, T. (2003). Read the archive and opening up the nation-state: Colonial knowledge in South Asia (and beyond). In A. Burton (Ed.), *After the imperial turn: Thinking with and through the nation* (pp. 102–121). Durham, NC: Duke University Press.

Barney, R. K. (1995). Studying stuff: Research in archives. In K. B. Wamsley (Ed.), *Method and methodology in sport and cultural history* (pp. 104–110). Dubuque, IA: Brown and Benchmark Publishers.

Berkhofer, R. (1995). *Beyond the great story: History as text and discourse*. Cambridge, MA: Harvard University Press.

Birrell, S., & Theberge, N. (1994). Ideological control of women in sport. In D. M. Costa & S. R. Guthrie (Eds.), *Women and Sport: Interdisciplinary Perspectives* (pp. 345–356). Champaign, IL: Human Kinetics.

Booth, D. (2005). *The field: Truth and fiction in sport history*. New York: Routledge.

Brown, D. (2007). The modern romance of mountaineering: Photography, aesthetics and embodiment. *International Journal of the History of Sport, 24*(1), 1–34.

Burke, P. (2001). *Eyewitnessing: The uses of images as historical evidence*. Ithaca, NY: Cornell University Press.

Burton, A. (2005). *Archive stories: Facts, fictions, and the writing of history*. Durham, NC: Duke University Press.

Cahn, S. K. (1994a). *Coming on strong: Gender and sexuality in twentieth-century women's sport*. Cambridge: Harvard University Press.

Cahn, S. K. (1994b). Sports talk: Oral history and its uses, problems, and possibilities for sport history. *The Journal of American History, 81*(2), 594–609.

Carr, E. H. (1969). *What is history?* Hampshire, UK: Palgrave Macmillan.

Cashman, R. (1995). *Paradise of sport: The rise of organised sport in Australia*. Melbourne: Oxford University Press.

Constanzo, M. (2002). One can't shake off the women: Images of sport and gender in punch 1901–10. *The International Journal of the History of Sport, 19*(1), 31–56.

Edwards, E., & Hart, J. (2004). *Photograph, objects, histories: On the materiality of images*. New York: Routledge.

Emery, L. (1994). From Lowell mills to the halls of fame: Industrial league sport for women. In D. M. Costa & S. R. Guthrie (Eds.), *Women and sport: Interdisciplinary perspectives* (pp. 107–121). Champaign, IL: Human Kinetics.

Fones-Wolf, E. (1986). Industrial recreation, the Second World War, and the revival of welfare capitalism, 1934–1960. *Business History Review, 60*, 232–257.

Forbes, S. L. (2001). Gendering corporate welfare practices: Female sports and recreation at Eaton's during the Depression. *Rethinking History, 5*(1), 59–74.

Franzosi, R. (1987). The press as source of socio-historical data: Issues in the methodology of data collection from newspapers. *Historical Methods, 20*(1), 5–16.

Fyfe, G., & Law, J. (1988). On the invisibility of the visual. In G. Fyfe & J. Law (Eds.), *Picturing power* (pp. 1–14). London: Routledge.

Gaskell, I. (1991). Visual history. In P. Burke (Ed.), *New perspectives in historical writing* (pp. 187–217). London: Polity.

Geiger, S. (1991). What's so feminist about women's oral history? *Journal of Women's History, 2*(1), 169–171.

Gems, G. R. (2001). Welfare capitalism and blue-collar sport: The legacy of labour unrest. *Rethinking History, 5*(1), 43–58.

Giardina, M., & Newman, J. (2011). Physical cultural studies and embodied research acts. *Cultural Studies ⇔ Critical Methodologies, 11*(6), 523–534.

Gleason, M. (1999). Embodied negotiations: Children's bodies and historical change in Canada, 1930–1960. *Journal of Canadian Studies, 34*(1), 112–138.

Guttmann, A. (1978). *From ritual to record: The nature of modern sports*. New York: Columbia University Press.

Hamilton, C., Harris, V., & Reid, G. (2002). Introduction. In C. Hamilton, V. Harris, J. Taylor, M. Pickover, G. Reid & R. Saleh (Eds.), *Refiguring the archive* (pp. 7–18). London: Kluwer Academic Publishers.

Hardy, S. (1982). *How Boston played: Sport, recreation and community, 1986–1915*. Boston, MA: Northeastern University Press.

Hargreaves, J. (1994). *Sporting females: Critical issues in the history and sociology of women's sports*. New York: Routledge.

Hargreaves, J., & Vertinsky, P. (2007). *Physical culture, power, and the body*. New York: Routledge.

Hill, J. (2006). Anecdotal evidence: Sport, the newspaper press, and history. In M. G. Phillips (Ed.), *Deconstructing sport history: A postmodern analysis* (pp. 117–130). Albany, NY: State University of New York Press.

Huggins, M. (2008). The sporting gaze: Towards a visual turn in sports history—Documenting art and sport. *Journal of Sport History, 35*(2), 311–329.

Huggins, M., & O'Mahony, M. (2011). Prologue: Extending study of the visual in the history of sport. *The International Journal of the History of Sport, 28*(8–9), 1089–1104.

Hunnicutt, B. K. (1996). *Kellogg's six-hour day*. Philadelphia, PA: Temple University Press.

Lenskyj, H. (1987). Physical activity for Canadian women, 1890–1930: Media views. In J. A. Mangan & R. J. Park (Eds.), *From 'fair sex' to feminism: Sport and the socialization of women in the industrial and post-industrial eras* (pp. 208–231). London, England: Frank Cass.

Metcalfe, A. (1987). *Canada learns to play: The emergence of organized sport, 1807–1914*. Toronto: McLelland & Stewart.

Munslow, A. (1997). *Reconstructing history*. London: Routledge.

O'Mahony, M. (2006). *Sport in the USSR: Physical culture – Visual culture*. London: Reaktion Books.

Oriard, M. (1993). *Reading football: How the popular press created an American spectacle*. Chapel Hill, NC: University of North Carolina Press.

Oriard, M. (2001). *King football: Sport & spectacle in the golden age of radio & newsreels, movies & magazines, the weekly & the daily Press*. Chapel Hill, NC: University of North Carolina Press.

Osmond, G. (2008). Reflecting materiality: Reading sport history through the lens. *Rethinking History, 12*(3), 339–360.

Osmond, G. (2010). Photographs, materiality and sport history: Peter Norman and the 1968 Mexico City black power salute. *Journal of Sport History*, *37*(1), 119–138.

Phillips, M. G. (2002). A critical appraisal of narrative in sport history: Reading the surf lifesaving debate. *Journal of Sport History*, *29*(1), 25–40.

Phillips, M. G., O'Neill, M. E., & Osmond, G. (2007). Broadening horizons in sport history: Films, photographs and monuments. *Journal of Sport History*, *34*(1), 271 293.

Portelli, A. (Ed.) (1991). What makes oral history different? In *The Death of Luigi Trastulli and Other Stories: Form and Meaning in Oral History* (pp. 45–58). New York: Oxford University Press.

Radar, B. (1983). *American sports: From the age of folk games to the age of spectators.* Englewood Cliffs, NJ: Prentice-Hall, Inc.

Rapley, T. (2004). Interviews. In C. Seale, G. Gabo, J. F. Gubrium & D. Silverman (Eds.), *Qualitative research practice* (pp. 15–33). Thousand Oaks, CA: Sage.

Rosenzweig, R. (1983). *Eight hours for what we will: Workers and leisure in an industrial city, 1870–1920*. New York: Cambridge University Press.

Sangster, J. (1993). The softball solution: Female workers, male managers and the operation of paternalism at Westclox, 1923–60. *Labour/Le Travail*, *32*, 167–199.

Sangster, J. (1995). *Earning respect: The lives of working women in small-town Ontario, 1920–1960*. Toronto: University of Toronto Press.

Sangster, J. (1997). Telling our stories: Feminist debates and the use of oral history. In V. Strong-Boag & A. C. Fellman (Eds.), *Rethinking Canada: The promise of women's history* (pp. 220–234). Toronto: Oxford University Press.

Schultz, J. (2006). Photography, instant memory and the slugging of Johnny Bright. *Stadion*, *32*, 221–243.

Stanford, M. (1994). *A companion to the study of history*. Oxford: Basil Blackwell.

Strong-Boag, V. (1979). The girl of the new day: Canadian working women in the 1920s. *Labour/Le Travail*, *4*, 132–163.

Struna, N. (2010). Historical research in physical activity. In J. R. Thomas, J. K. Nelson, S. Silverman & S. J. Silverman (Eds.), *Research methods in physical activity* (pp. 217–234). Champaign, IL: Human Kinetics.

Thomson, A. (1998). Fifty years on: An international perspective on oral history. *The Journal of American History*, *85*(2), 581–595.

Thompson, P. (2000). *The voice of the past: Oral history*. New York: Oxford University Press.

Thyssen, G. (2007). Visualizing discipline of the body in a German open-air school (1923–1939): Retrospection and introspection. *Journal of the History of Education Society*, *36*(2), 247–264.

White, H. (1973). *Metahistory: The historical imagination in 19th century Europe*. Baltimore, MD: John Hopkins University Press.

Yacob, S. (2008). Model of welfare capitalism: The United States rubber company in Southeast Asia, 1910–1942. *Enterprise and Society*, *8*(1), 136–176.

Zahavi, G. (1998). *Workers, managers and welfare capitalism*. Urbana, IL: University of Illinois Press.

CHAPTER 2

THE EMPIRICAL STRIKES BACK: DOING REALIST ETHNOGRAPHY

Michael Atkinson

ABSTRACT

Purpose – This chapter explores a traditional mode of ethnography referred to as 'realist ethnography' as it relates to sport and physical culture (SPC) research.

Design/methodology/approach – The chapter discusses different approaches to ethnography, but principally addresses a realist ethnography I conducted on Ashtanga yoga in Canada.

Findings – I discuss how data evolved from the realist ethnographic method, and outline the manner in which ethnographic research is as a 'way of life'. The chapter concludes that the realist ethnographic method is not untenable, as some authors suggest, but rather a viable and exciting mode of knowledge production in the SPC field.

Originality/value – The chapter is original work. It makes a case for the retention of realist ethnographies in our methodological lexicon, and illustrates the empirical process of writing culture. It also endeavours to

Qualitative Research on Sport and Physical Culture
Research in the Sociology of Sport, Volume 6, 23–49
Copyright © 2012 by Emerald Group Publishing Limited
All rights of reproduction in any form reserved
ISSN: 1476-2854/doi:10.1108/S1476-2854(2012)0000006005

engage students and scholars alike regarding the value of ethnographic methods more broadly.

Keywords: Ethnography; realism; participant observation; fieldwork; Ashtanga yoga

INTRODUCTION

Once the staple method of qualitative researchers across North America and elsewhere, *ethnography* (often referred to as 'field research', 'participant observation' or 'naturalistic inquiry') is the study of human group life via a researcher's immersion in a particular social group, (sub)culture, scene or cultural setting of interest. An ethnographer becomes a participant in, and in many cases a full-fledged member of, a group to study its everyday workings, to learn what the culture means to its members, to grasp how it shapes members' worldviews and life practices, and to conceptualise how cultural life is organised and exercised. Some ethnographers link micrological studies of cultural life to macro social trends and process (e.g. globalisation, political economic forces, institutional structures of inequality and power), while many focus on how cultural mores provide maps of meaning for people in the 'here and now' of everyday life. In this chapter, I review the logic and practices of performing classical, realist ethnography with specific reference to an extended fieldwork project on Ashtanga Vinyasa Yoga in Canada. I discuss an array of the 'ins' and 'outs' of performing realist ethnography, and highlight a range of topics, problems and opportunities typically ignored or downplayed in garden-variety dissections of the method.

REALIST ETHNOGRAPHIC ENCOUNTERS

My ethnographic research on Ashtanga yoga commenced in 2005. As a woefully inflexible recreational athlete, I started practising Ashtanga yoga (hereafter, simply referred to as *Ashtanga*) as a complementary strength and recovery technique to my running, duathlon and triathlon adventures. Ashtanga is an ancient brand of yoga derived from the *Yoga Sutras of Patanjali* and the *Yoga Korunta*. The practice of an Ashtanga 'session' focuses on generating heat in the body through a set of prescribed bending, balancing and strength-building postures (called *asanas*), deep and cleansing breathing, and meditation. Like other forms of yoga in Canada, Ashtanga's popularity has grown almost exponentially since the 1990s. Where one might have been hard-pressed to locate an Ashtanga studio in most Canadian urban environments in the early 1990s, options now abound.

Almost immediately after commencing my Ashtanga practice at a small studio in Hamilton, Ontario, in 2005, I researched much deeper into 'Ashtangi' culture in Canada. I moved away from the study while working in the United Kingdom, only to resume it after returning to Canada in the summer of 2009. In the autumn of 2009, I stumbled across a 'traditional' Ashtanga studio in Toronto (traditional studios are called *shalas*) and dove deeply into an ethnographic foray on the subject. In what follows, I outline my preferences and predilections for realist ethnography as a methodological vehicle for grasping/theorising the Ashtanga culture I study in Toronto, and how such traditional ethnographic modes of inquiry are arguably foundational qualitative techniques for knowing the lived experiences of cultural others. But before walking through my research in this chapter, definitional matters regarding the concept of realist ethnography warrant time and space.

So ... Just What is [Realist] Ethnography, Anyway?

The term ethnography (from the Greek *ethnos*, meaning 'people', and *graph*, meaning 'writing') itself is quite loosely and lazily applied to *any* qualitative research project where observation of others is used to provide an inductive, detailed, in-depth description of the everyday-life practices of a group of people. This is sometimes referred to (and, again, haphazardly) as a 'thick description' of culture – a term attributed to the cultural anthropologist Clifford Geertz (1973). Realist ethnographers generate blended substantive and theoretical understandings of culture through systematic analyses of multiple insiders' points of view. A realist ethnographer believes that in order to understand, translate and conceptually explain how cultures function, and how they provide what Raymond Williams (1977) describes as 'maps of meaning' for people, one needs to become a member of that culture. Theoretical knowledge about cultures is best generated, a realist ethnographic epistemology upholds, by direct contact and experience with members of a culture over time. Therefore, the epistemology is straightforward; one becomes a member of a cultural group, does what they do, travels with them and lives alongside them as a means of achieving intersubjectivity with them.

Robert Prus (1996), building on a Chicago-style symbolic interactionist approach to qualitative research as informed by George Herbert Mead, Herbert Blumer and Carl Couch, argues that the role of the realist ethnographer is to explore and theorise the origins, meanings and production of the *generic social processes* (GSPs) structuring human group life. GSPs refer to ubiquitous processes constituting group life such as developing cultural perspectives, engaging in the cultural activities with others, achieving identity in groups, forming relationships with people and forming commitments to cultural communities. Ethnographers adopt a realist epistemology to develop nuanced and complex theoretical understandings GSPs from the 'ground up'; emphasis is thus placed on allowing abstract concepts and meanings about the GSPs in our social worlds to *emerge* from the ethnographic encounter rather than imposing these from existing theoretical models.

In the end, realist ethnographic research provides a representational (usually written) account of a particular culture during a specified time period. After spending time 'in the field' with the people and mapping their culture, the ethnographer crafts an interpretivist account of the culture and what it is like to be shaped as a person by the culture. Such accounts are described as *realist depictions* (Prus, 1996) of social life. *Realism* refers to the notion that ethnographers feel confident in telling 'reality-congruent' (Elias, 1987) sociological stories about groups under study following long-term involvement with them. Stated differently, after a long period of sympathetic introspection in the field living shoulder to shoulder with others, one is able to *know* and be able to *sociologically capture* their life worlds in intimate, intersubjective detail. After fully immersing into the culture over time, a realist ethnographer feels confident enough that s/he is able to write an account of the culture that accurately represents its core values, structures, processes and participants. Therefore, if you wish to sociologically study a particular physical cultural practice like golfing or snowboarding, you become a golfer or a snowboarder and hang around with others immersed in the practice. But how any ethnographic venture is conducted, how data are analysed and the use of ethnographic data are far more complex matters.

Realist ethnographic methods have been employed quite extensively in studies of sport, physical culture and leisure over the past thirty years (Atkinson, 2011). To name only a few, ethnographic efforts on the analysis of surfers (Sands, 2001), boxers (Wacquant, 2004), skateboarders (Beal,

1995), snowboarders (Thorpe, 2011), sport for development volunteer workers (Darnell, 2010), NASCAR fans (Newman & Giardina, 2011), windsurfers (Wheaton, 2000), media production workers (Silk, 2001), rugby players (Howe, 2001) and bodybuilders (Monaghan, 2001) have all been produced. In my own research, I have employed ethnographic methods to study diverse groups including duathletes and triathletes, traceurs, fell runners, greyhound racing enthusiasts, anorexics in sport and, most recently, youth sport coaches in Canada. Sport and physical culture (SPC) researchers undertake modes of ethnography to address questions pertaining to who participates in sport, how sport is a site for the (re)production of identities (gender, race, class, ethnicity, sexuality, religious), how sport involvement is shaped by one's geographic and historical space/place and how small-group resistance to prevailing social norms, values, discourses and institutional structures may be waged through sport and physical cultural participation (Atkinson & Young, 2008).

Realist ethnographies involve the close exploration of several sources of data 'in the field'. First and foremost, long-term engagement in the field setting or place where people in the culture meet and interact daily is essential and most commonly called *participant observation*. This is perhaps the primary source of ethnographic data, and the term is often conflated with the term ethnography itself. The notion of participant observation captures the dual role of the ethnographer in that one is both a participant in the culture, but at the same time is an academic observer. Elias (1987) outlines the degree to which a (field) researcher, like any other social scientist, must strive towards maintaining a balance between empirical involvement with subjects (required to gain a sympathetic understanding of others) and cognitive/emotional detachment from them (required to sociologically recognise the conceptual themes, patterns and structures – or GSPs – organising everyday life). To develop an involved/detached understanding of what it is like to be a member of a culture, the researcher becomes a *participant* in the life of the settings wherein the culture operates, while also maintaining the stance of an *observer*, someone who can describe the experience with a measure of what we might call professional detachment. Note that this does not prevent ethnographers from becoming advocates for the people they study (in particular, see John Sugden's discussion of investigative sociology and research ethics in Chapter 11).

Realist ethnographers typically spend many months or even years conducting field research, often forming lasting bonds with people there. To be sure, many undergraduate students, graduate students and faculty members conduct ethnographies in the communities where they themselves

(margin handwritten note: Ethnographers – study people in natural setting & become one of them. Observe/participate unknowingly)

live and work. Gold (1958) describes four principal ways in which people become ethnographically emplaced in a community to conduct research. These participatory roles range along a continuum of involvement, from complete participant (one who is fully immersed and participates in the culture) to participant as observer (one who participates, but not in everything), to observer as participant (one who moderately participates, but principally watches the culture from the social periphery), to complete observer (one who observers the culture only, without ever participating in or interacting among its members).

At some point in time, most ethnographers will also interview members of the culture or setting under study in order to deepen their understandings of the people there, and to collect life history data on the group's members. Thus, realist ethnographic methods are undertaken quite frequently as triangulation-based studies. Ethnographic interviews provide a context for focused data collection by asking specific but open-ended questions among key informants identified through the research process. There is a great variety of interview styles, and each ethnographer brings his or her own unique approach to the process. Regardless, the emphasis is on allowing the person or persons being interviewed to answer without being limited by pre-defined choices – something which clearly differentiates qualitative from more quantitative or demographic approaches. In most cases, an ethnographic interview looks and feels little different than an everyday conversation and indeed in the course of long-term participant-observation, most ethnographic conversations are in fact purely spontaneous and without any specific agenda. Researchers collect other sources of data that depend on the specific nature of the field setting. This may take the form of representative artefacts that embody characteristics of the topic of interest, government reports, and newspaper and magazine articles. Although often not tied to the site of study, secondary academic sources are utilised to locate the specific study within an existing body of literature.

(ALTERNATIVE) MODELS AND STRATEGIES FOR DEVELOPING ETHNOGRAPHIC RESEARCH PROJECTS

Aside from the realist ethnographic method described above, there is any number of ethnographic modes of inquiry at the disposal of a researcher. Throughout the first three quarters of the twenty-first century, the lion's share of ethnographic inquiries displayed realist orientation. Following a progressive scepticism regarding an ethnographer's ability to merely represent the 'objective' aspects of social/cultural life via a textual account of others (see Denzin, 2003; Gubrium & Holstein, 1997), a panorama of ethnographic forms emerged that privilege polysemic, fractured and radically contextual social constructions of cultural realities. Newer (and now more popular than realist) modes of ethnography include standpoint, queer, post-structural and postmodern, feminist, institutional, auto-ethnographic, media, audience, internet-based, sensory, mobile, visual, blitzkrieg, guerrilla and others (Atkinson, 2011). It is beyond the scope of this chapter to enumerate differences between all ethnographic modes, but a handful is worth highlighting.

A number of research questions are well suited for the family of ethnographic approaches. By and large, though, research questions focusing on the ways in which membership in certain social groups or cultures shape one's personal and collective sport and physical cultural practices are most amenable to ethnographic modes of inquiry. For example, my first fully ethnographic venture homed in on the ticket scalping subculture in Toronto, Canada (Atkinson, 2000). I wanted to know how the subculture is (re)produced, how members are brought in, how tickets are acquired and what this illegal subculture signifies with regard to the broader sports-entertainment complex in Canada. Such is a classic example of a (sub)*cultural ethnography*. The purpose of these ethnographies is to learn the inner workings of a very small group/subculture and then explain how and why the culture operates as it does, inductively, as a theoretical venture. Ethnographies involving the study of two or more groups/cultures over time are often called *ethnologies*, while historical accounts of a culture arising from a study of them are referred to as *ethnohistories*. Although not a prerequisite of small-scale cultural ethnography, researchers will occasionally strive to connect what is learned in a local cultural setting with broader trends and processes in a society (Wolcott, 1999). In my ticket scalping study, I argued that the scalping subculture itself is partially produced by diffuse market capitalist trends in sport and elsewhere.

Institutional ethnography is an increasingly popular ethnographic approach to empirical inquiry associated with the feminist scholar Dorothy Smith (1987). The approach emphasises connections among the sites and situations of everyday life, professional practice and policy making. Smith (1987) developed the approach initially from a feminist perspective, calling it a method that could produce a sociology for women; yet, she describes it as an approach with much wider application. In essence, an institutional

ethnography (sometimes called *standpoint ethnography*) strives to understand how people's everyday lives are structured by social forces working
through and within institutions like the family, media, workplaces, schools
and others. Those following Smith in the development of institutional
ethnographic methods have taken up a variety of substantive topics, including the organisation of health care, education, social work practice, the
regulation of sexuality, the police and the judicial processing of violence
against women, employment and job training, economic and social rest-
ructuring, international development regimes, planning and environmental
policy, the organisation of home and community life, and various kinds of
activism. To date, and quite surprisingly, very few SPC researchers have
explored the potential of institutional or standpoint ethnography (though
many have engaged a version of institutional ethnography more loosely
described as *feminist ethnography*).

More recently, *auto-ethnographic* methods have grown in popularity
within the study of sport, physical activity and health. Auto-ethnography
is a method in which the investigator develops a research question
pertaining to a particular social process, experience or reality and then
creates an ethnographic description and analysis of his/her own behaviour,
attempting to develop an objective understanding of the behaviours and
work context under consideration by casting the investigator as both the
informant 'insider' and the analyst 'outsider'. For example, a spate of
running auto-ethnographies has been published within the recent past
(Hockey, 2006). These ethnographies, almost always written in a story or
aesthetic narrative form rather than as a traditional academic/journal
article, illustrate that by knowing one's own self and exploring how one's
own life takes meaning (for instance, as a runner), we learn a great deal
about the processes by which social life unfolds. Auto-ethnographies can
be deeply personal, emotional and artistic in their written form, as part of
the logic of the method is to 'open up' and personalise published research
in order to help readers connect with academic arguments, theories and
ideas (see Chapter 9).

Audience ethnography strives to understand how people actively receive,
decode and use media texts. Audience ethnography might be designed as a
one-shot case study, or be structured as a long-term panel study of how a
group interprets media over the course of time. In the typical scenario,
participants in an audience ethnographic project are asked to collectively or
individually watch, read or listen to selected media and then respond to its
content. A researcher acts as a facilitator in these scenarios, prompting
questions among respondents about what the messages or symbols in the

media might mean to them and how they actively decode them from a variety of cultural standpoints (age, race, sexuality, gender, class). The underpinning logic of doing audience ethnography is that by observing and questioning how people make sense of media data 'live' and *in situ*, researchers compile a more valid understanding of the process of immediate reception and the cognitive processing of media content. Wilson and Sparks (1996), for example, illustrate how African Canadian teenage boys fashion their own constructions of, and lived experiences with, Black masculinity to interpret mass mediations of 'Blackness' in basketball shoe advertisements. Wilson and Sparks (1996) discuss how the boys find humour, reality and frequent inferential racism in the depictions of Black masculinity in the advertisements. They also attest to how the youth selectively take from the commercials what makes sense to them culturally, and how they negate or resist supposedly preferred images and constructions of 'Blackness' in the commercials.

A relatively new mode of ethnographic inquiry, *sensory ethnography*, is described by sociologist Sarah Pink (2009) as a way of thinking about and doing ethnography that takes, as its starting point, the multisensoriality (hearing, seeing, smelling, tasting and touching) essence of human experience, perception, knowing and practice. Pink describes sensory ethnography as an outcropping of a traditional form of ethnography, that further accounts for how people's experiences with multisensoriality in social life is integral both to the lives of people who participate in our research and to how ethnographers practice field methods. A number of ethnographers have begun to comment on the multisensoriality of the ethnographic process, including scholars who study SPC like Larry de Garis (1999) whose work has focused on understanding the sensory/sensuous aspects of professional wrestling.

Performance (or 'performative') ethnography is an emerging arts-based method of qualitative inquiry and representation that presents a tangible opportunity to bridge the gap between scholarly activity and community teaching and learning. After spending time in the field with a group of normally marginalised others, the ethnographer, generally in conjunction with key informants from the group under study, writes and produces a dramatic play, vignette or short film representing the culture. By using the theatre or the screen as a place of research representation, performance ethnography transforms them from a place of entertainment to a venue for participatory action research that extends beyond the performance itself (Alexander, 2005; Finley, 2005; Kemmis & McTaggart, 2005). As a forum for cultural exchange, the power of performance ethnography lies in its

potential for illumination and engagement of involved researchers, participants and audience.

Finally, with the rise of new online media, the practice of *netnography* is
gaining popularity as a technique of analysis. Netnography, or online
ethnography, is literally an online ethnography of Internet sites wherein a
researcher does not simply observe the content of websites, but often
contributes to them as a registered or recognised member. Wilson and
Atkinson (2005), for example, studied the online recruiting and social
connecting mechanisms provided by Rave and Straightedge blogs and chat
forums/rooms. In both subcultures, youth in these respective physical
cultures use Internet sites as a performing community and a way of fostering
bonds between members across great spaces. Both of the researchers
participated and chatted with members online as a means of conducting
quasi-interviews, but, more importantly, of gaining a first-hand understanding of how new media space is produced by groups in 'real time' as a
vehicle for developing a sense of mutual identification and commitment.
Whatever the form of ethnography one adopts, the epistemological core of
the approach remains somewhat constant. Ethnography translates into the
pursuit of socio-cultural knowledge about the world from the places, spaces,
contexts, processes and fields in which it is performed from day to day.
Ethnographers (generally) believe that rather than applying theoretical
assumptions *a priori* about the meaning, significance and experience of life
to cultural cases studies before actually engaging with people, theorising is
best accomplished via sustained engagement with actors 'out there' in one
context or another.

'OM BOY': A REALIST ETHNOGRAPHY OF ASHTANGA

An ethnography is neither an academic project one participates in a leisurely
fashion nor a hobby undertaken in one's spare-time spectrum. Full-scale,
realist ethnographies totally encompass and connect one's professional and
personal lives. This is the essential, and critical, logic of the method.
Ethnographers tend to believe in generating theory through experiential
education; that is, seeing, doing and feeling first-hand is the best pathway to
believing, knowing and theorising sociologically. Although a contested
argument, a realist ethnographer might only 'truly' know a culture after one
perceives him/herself to be a practising member of said culture. When one

achieves roles, statuses and identities in the culture; views themselves as a member of the culture and shares a commitment to the reproduction of the culture, ethnographic modes of knowing are shifted into high gear. Ethnographies require time, patience, energy, and the willingness to immerse physically, socially, cognitively and emotionally in others' cultures. When one chooses to study sport and physical cultural worlds ethnographically, one's entire modality of living shifts. For this reason alone, neophyte ethnographers must reflexively analyse their own enthusiasm for social interaction with strangers, their ability to manage interpersonal stage fright, their desire to spend copious amounts of time away from friends and family members and their capability for sacrificing almost all of their free time.

Being an Ashtangi is arduous for many reasons. Firstly, there are two essential 'paths' (sadhanas) one follows in traditional Ashtanga culture: the total devotee who abandons all else to pursue the practice, and the 'householder' – the common John or Sally who has a family, career, friends outside of yoga but who wishes to practice Ashtanga nevertheless. And yes, Ashtanga yoga is a *total practice* of/for living. I once believed that Ashtanga simply refereed to a set of traditional exercises performed in discrete time blocks of 60 to 90 minutes per day. In the *Yoga Sutras*, however, Patanjali writes that the two core principles for practising yoga are *abhyasa* (devotion, or single focus on practice) and *vairagya* (non-attachment). Abhyasa means having an attitude of persistent effort (a physical, mental and emotional practice) to attain and maintain a state of stable tranquility (equanimity). To become well established, this needs to be done for a long time, without a break – it means, in the first instance, practising asana (poses) six days a week, every week, without fail. Vairagya is the essential companion of non-attachment; learning to let go of the many attachments, aversions, fears and false identities that Ashtangis believe are clouding the true, and eternal, self.

The term Ashtanga, itself, is a composite of the Sanskrit words 'ashta' meaning 'eight', and 'anga' meaning 'limb'. The practice of Ashtanga is an eight-fold path – distilled differently, there are eight steps or limbs for doing abhyasa leading to vairagya. After learning about the core principles early on in my ethnography (which simply formed around the question of 'What it is like to be a member of an Ashtanga yogic culture?'), I knew this could not be a physical culture I participated in 'lightly' if I was to truly understand its meaning and significance to practitioners. The limbs or steps in the path relate to the principles for achieving enlightenment as outlined in the Yoga Sutras. Each limb is essential in 'practising' Ashtanga, and there is logical order to how they must be approached. Respectively, the eight limbs are *Yama* (five moral restraints – non-violence, truthfulness, control of the senses, non-stealing and non-covetousness); *Niyama* (five observances – purity, contentment, austerity, study of scriptures and surrender to God's will); *Asana* (postures); *Pranayama* (breath control); *Pratyahara* (withdrawal of the senses); *Dharana* (concentration); *Dhyana* (meditation) and *Samadhi* (a super-conscious state).

I have always found that ethnographies centring on a 'main' physical cultural practice like yoga are easier to initiate than those involving a heterogeneous group doing heterogeneous things. In truth, SPC ethnographies almost always congeal around a central practice of sport, leisure or activity. With respect to the daily physical practice of asana (my entrance or access point into the culture), Ashtanga is different physical culture from many other yoga systems and styles now popular in the West. The order of asanas during one's daily is completely predefined. This proved to be somewhat comforting during my early days in the field at 'The Ashtanga House' in Toronto. In the early days, most ethnographic work is harrowing. Managing stage fright in front of others, feeling awkward in new settings, finding a place to meet people in the culture and finding a role to legitimate one's presence there are tasks one encounters. Because there are fewer than a handful of 'traditional' Ashtanga shalas in Toronto, and because the shala space is defined by set patterns of interaction that include, as a regular course of cultural practice, newcomers, I felt at ease in the setting from the onset.

My first six months in the shala followed the same routine. I think finding a routine and settling into an interactive 'groove' in the field puts an ethnographer at ease quickly, and allows one to culturally acclimatise to the surroundings. For many weeks, I simply kept my eyes and ears open, and my mouth shut. I observed a lot, met a few people in the change rooms, started speaking with the studio director and head teacher at The Ashtanga House ('Darren') and learned the poses. This was my ethnographic work for the first six months of the study; being there on a regular basis, learning the asana sequence, watching everything and writing as many field notes as possible in a notebook while sitting in my car after every practice.

Ashtanga is traditionally taught in 'Mysore style' (supervised self-practice, and named after the city in India where Ashtanga originates) at The Ashtanga House. Mysore style involves students moving through the practice at their own pace and level. The Ashtanga House in Toronto opens daily at 5:45 am and Mysore practice runs until 1:30 pm with the exception of Saturdays (the prescribed one day off during the week). Mysore style is the traditional method of learning the practice, in which an individual is progressively 'given' poses from an Ashtanga series by a teacher when the student is ready to receive them. One may enter the main Mysore practice room in a shala like the one at The Ashtanga House in Toronto at any time during the morning session, and commence the asanas one has received to date. My teacher, Darren, oversees Mysore practice every morning (after doing his own asana practice at home at 3:30 am) along with two to three of his assistants who aid students with physical alignment in particularly problematic postures. The Mysore room is stiflingly hot, humid, dimly lit, sweat soaked, packed with bodies and deathly quiet. The only audible sounds are feet hitting the mats at points and heavy, deep nasal breathing from practitioners. An individual with an established Ashtanga practice might take between an hour and two hours to complete Mysore-style practice in the morning, depending on his or her own personal level and experience.

The Ashtanga practice of asana comprises four main parts: an opening sequence, one of the six main 'series' of poses, a back bending sequence and a set of inverted asanas referred to as the 'finishing sequence'. The opening sequence begins with ten Sun Salutations and then several standing asanas. Next, the practitioner will do one of the six main series – the Primary series ('Yoga Chikitsa'), Intermediate series ('Nadi Shodhana') or Advanced A, B, C or D ('Sthira Bhaga'). Newcomers to Ashtanga practise the Primary series under the watchful eye of the shala's main teacher, Darren. Practitioners advance to more difficult series over a period of years or decades.

The sheer demand of a daily practice constantly reminded me of the absolute centrality of 'being there' as part of the realist ethnographic method. Daily or regular practice is strongly encouraged in Ashtanga culture as a means of taking the first steps to pursuing abhyasa. I knew, from very early on in the ethnography, that my entire style of life would need reorganisation for me to pursue this ethnography. Why? In order for me to practice, I needed to manage the following: fitting daily practice into a schedule packed with work commitments, family responsibilities (escorting my sons to and from school, spending time with my family etc.), friendship duties, long-standing eating and sleeping habits, and other competing physical practices like running and cycling. I intuitively knew the answers to each of these realist ethnographic dilemmas. I had to practice asanas at 6:00 am before work, get to bed by 8:30 pm most evenings, never eat after 6:00 pm (Ashtangis believe in practising on an empty stomach), convincing my wife to support my practice and assume my morning childcare duties, relinquishing other research projects and university-related responsibilities, culling my circle of friends outside of the culture for some time and neglecting my running and cycling practices. Ashtanga, like any other physical culture, can be a demanding, jealous mistress. A realist ethnographer quickly learns that competing interests do not fare well in the progress of one's research.

By late 2010, I had fully immersed into an Ashtangi lifestyle. I learned to hate the sound of my alarm clock, felt perpetually 'hung over' for weeks to the rigours of the practice, felt my body change considerably, developed close friendships with a core group of people at the shala and did whatever I could to participate in different aspects of the culture emanating from the studio, such as workshops, a 100-hour immersion course and shala-organised social events. After my evening bedtime story rituals with my two sons, I spent most nights reading yogic texts and sutras. Nearly a half-dozen of my full diaries of field notes and 200 magazine articles filled a filing cabinet in my office. Everyone at the shala came to know me as 'Mike, the guy from the university studying yoga'. My modality of living changed dramatically, and I increasingly found it difficult to squeeze the rest of my life into the study. Then, and only then, was I confident of my full immersion in Ashtanga culture. The physical culture had become 'real' in my life, structuring my daily activities, thoughts and relationships; this is the methodological cornerstone of the notion of 'real' in realist ethnography.

Doing It 'By the Book'

The ethnographic research I conducted on Ashtanga is my first serious attempt at performing realist ethnography 'by the book'. While I have completed a half-dozen ethnographic projects in the last fifteen years, this is the first long-term ethnographic research project I have undertaken in accordance with the core procedural guidelines for realist ethnography.

First, realist ethnography is the process of knowing a subject by *doing and becoming through immersed observation*. Very early in my training as sociologist, I developed a particular fascination with techniques for learning culture by experiencing it moving and being shaped in the field. Rather than studying social interaction through a detached or quasi-objective position, I firmly believe in learning about a subject by social immersion in it. This is, of course, not possible in all contexts of sociological inquiry, but in the case of Ashtanga, I have been fully immersed in the practice for nearly three years. Realist ethnographies are predicated on one's ability to be situated, in context, for extended periods of time. To me, there is no greater ethnographic commitment to knowing how others frame and experience culture, than through persistent emplacement (physical, emotional, cognitive, and identity and role based) in a culture.

Second, the persistent immersion process allows for sociological discovery. Paul Willis (1998) writes that the greatest benefit of sustained ethnographic participation and social observation is that we routinely are 'surprised' by what people are actually doing, saying and feeling in their lives. We may begin, for instance, to challenge our own taken-for-granted (or commonsense) sociological claims about the world by taking the roles of many others. My research program on Ashtanga congealed into a long-term, theoretically open-ended venture aimed at exploring many of the taken-for-granted truths about dominant and alternative physical cultural practices. As discussed below in further detail, this meant suspending, to the best of my ability, my learned academic tendencies to theoretically 'direct' an ethnographic investigation (or presuppose one's findings) by comfortable, favoured or avant-garde concepts from the outset of research.

Third, realist ethnography is a process of living among and working with people as a means of *knowledge production through story telling*. I spend copious amounts of time in the field listening to stories people tell about their lived experiences with Ashtanga. I juxtapose these against my own personal stories and lived experiences with the physical culture, and weave them together to form preliminary theoretical understandings of the practice. Despite any claim otherwise, realist ethnography *has always been* focused on the co-production (researcher/subjects) of accounts (or stories) about life. Here, researchers learn, discuss, work with and share stories from others in the field in order to, in the end, represent a sociological story about a physical culture like Ashtanga.

Fourth, when our stories have been gathered and collated, and typically condensed into one main (meta)narrative, *truth claims* about the world are woven together into conceptual abstractions. Strategies of analytic induction are especially beneficial in realist ethnography. Here is where, at least for me, one of the most contentious and misunderstood aspects of realist ethnography creeps into the methodological frame. Traditional inductive work in realist ethnography is generally referred to as the pursuit of *grounded theory*. For me, this an academic hallmark of realist ethnographic work. Grounded theory is perhaps most accurately described as an inductive research technique in which the eventual theory one 'discovers' about the nature of social/cultural life is developed from the data, rather than the other way around. Data collection, analysis and theory formulation are undeniably connected in a reciprocal sense, and the 'grounded theory' approach incorporates explicit procedures to guide this process (see

Charmaz, 2003; Glaser, 2001; Strauss & Corbin, 1998). Doing grounded theory is, at once, a process of collecting data, interpreting data, developing conceptual ideas and eventually developing formal hypotheses about the nature of social reality in a particular group (or potentially across groups) under study.

A grounded theoretical approach in realist ethnography has the potential to shed new, innovative, challenging and paradigm-directing insights on the nature of social reality(ies). For example, I pursued a theoretically grounded study of Ashtanga, pursued not so I merely become a substantive expert on the physical culture itself (which invariably happens) but so that the systematic study of Ashtanga culture may teach me about GSPs, conditions, features or aspects of the human group experience. Some argue that this approach borders on sociological metaphysics, and that ethnographic researchers should eschew the pursuit of any notion of a theoretical universal when it comes to studying lived experience.

While debates regarding the proper application of the method abound, I believe there is no other approach to ethnographic data analysis as well suited for generating creative theoretical insight on world. But academics are funny, and in many ways very predictable, creatures of habit. I have spent the better part of the last twenty years developing my own theoretical tastes and preferences for reading social reality – around questions of human agency, power, suffering, exploitation, structuration and so forth. My previous theoretical penchants for concepts from figurational sociology, Marxist-leaning cultural studies perspectives or central tenets of symbolic interaction had to be avoided at the outset of my research. Concepts from these theoretical traditions are not, technically, allowed to surface in a 'grounded' study of mine on Ashtanga.

I had to avoid the trap of conflating the pursuit of grounded theory with guided theoretical induction, or what I have referred to elsewhere (Atkinson, 2011) as qualitative *concept elaboration*. In doing concept elaboration (which is by most erroneously referred to as grounded theoretical development), a researcher commences with a set of pre-configured conceptual ideas in mind (or their preferred theoretical explanations of the world), and then applies them to emergent qualitative data as a means of hermeneutically 'reading', sorting and classifying the cultural practices under investigation. It is research produced, directed, represented and received through the lens of pre-existing concepts. The concepts might be expanded, contracted, tightened or partially redefined through the ethnographic inquiry, but rarely are new theoretical ideas, concepts or entire meta-theories produced.

Proper grounded theory in a realist ethnographic venture is a general research method which guides researchers on matters of data collection (where you can use data of any type – e.g. video, images, text, observations, and spoken word) and details strict procedures for data analysis. In a much more 'academic' sounding definition, grounded theory is a research tool enabling one to seek out and conceptualise the latent cultural patterns and human experiences in a setting under study through the process of *constant comparison* (a fancy term describing the 'constant' interpretation of emerging data in a study with every bit of data collected beforehand). How does the method unfold in practice? In my ethnographic research on Ashtanga, I adopted the following steps to pursue a grounded theoretical reading of the culture:

1. Identification of the substantive area, or the discrete cultural groups to be studied. In my research, I chose to study a relatively small (approximately 120) group of people who regularly attend a very traditional Ashtanga shala in north Toronto.
2. Collection of data pertaining to the substantive area. Realist ethnographies begin, and continue for years at times, as open-ended inquires with only very loosely defined research questions. Data collection is, therefore, expansive, opportunistic, all-encompassing and never ending. In my research, data collection includes the following:
    o Going to daily practice at the shala, attending workshops and retreats, and participating in Ashtanga conferences in Canada;
    o Reading nearly two-dozen published books about Ashtanga yoga, hundreds of magazine articles, watching on-line videos and reading blogs, and joining social media sites devoted to the practice.
    o Conversing with individuals (informally, or through interviews) or a group of individuals about Ashtanga. For me, this involved hundreds of hours of socialisation with Ashtangis and conducting thirty-seven interviews with instructors and practitioners.
3. 'Open coding' the above data as I collected it in small waves. Open coding and data collection in realist ethnography are integrated activities throughout a study; thus, the data collection stage and open coding stage occur simultaneously and continue until a core theoretical idea or concept is recognised and selected as the focus of research. This coding occurred across, and simultaneously with, all aspects of my data collection on Ashtanga: from personal Mysore practice to interviews, to reading, to website analysis, to *in situ* observations and so forth. Open coding is the first step in reducing the 'volume' of data in a study like mine, and

identifying sociological 'things' happening the culture. No textbook can, in honesty, teach someone how to open code. An open code is an idea, really, that you believe conceptually captures something you saw, heard or experienced. Here, you are not simply applying a well-worn sociological concept (like anomie, or norms, or alienation) to something you have observed, but rather coming up with potentially new codes/labels that emerge from your field study. An open code is simply something you write down in a field journal, or in the margins of an interview transcript as a way of sociologically classifying what you are observing. Becoming skilled at opening coding is more art than science, relying on one's ability to use reason, logic, intuition, empathy, intersubjectivity, affect and wisdom to 'see' sociological things in the culture you are immersed in as research. This is perhaps why, I feel, so many contemporary field researchers prefer concept elaboration as the method of ethnographic analysis over a proper grounded theoretical approach.

4. After a while, a realist ethnographer conducts selective coding and theoretical sampling in a study like mine. In all likelihood, one or two major 'open codes' will become the focus of your investigation. In my study of Ashtanga, I open coded a litany of field observations, interviewee quotes, personal experiences and excerpts from blogs and readings as *retrenchment*. It, along with several others, developed into what is normally called a 'core [conceptual] category'. When I began to see the theme of retrenchment in my data, it developed into what one might call a main sociological concern – or, in other terms, it emerged as a core research question in the study. At this point, open coding across my data stopped, and 'selective coding' – coding only for the core categories – began. Basically, what happens is that you begin to dive deeper into the dimensions or rungs or sub-categories of the emerging 'concept'. For example, I sub-coded forms of retrenchment as retrenchment from the mental self, the body, an array of cultural practices, particular social identities, structurally conditioned ways of living and so forth. From there, I purposefully focused my field observations, interviews and readings on retrenchment activities in Ashtanga. I interviewed people with specific knowledge about the different dimensions of retrenchment, and started thinking about what, at this particular time in our Canadian history, might be leading people to seek Ashtanga yoga as a means/ vehicle for retrenchment.

5. Once I felt I was learning relatively little that was 'new' about retrenchment from my ethnography (referred to as the stage of data saturation), it was appropriate to search for and attempt to integrate

sociological literature(s) about retrenchment with my existing research on Ashtanga.

Traditional grounded theory is more of an interpretive art rather than a science. I know of no template, manual, set of tactical procedures or foolproof steps for conducting grounded theory in a realist ethnography. There are recommendations, canons and principles, but one simply cannot be taught how to code, interpret and generate new concepts or even a new theory with the requisite degree of creativity needed to flourish in the practice. University courses, seminars and workshops abound as means of exposing researchers to the principles of grounded theory, but analytic flair cannot be learned in the classroom. Perhaps, this is why I have avoided pure grounded theoretical work until quite recently. Neophytes to the approach often find the entire procedure vexing and inaccessible as a data collection and analysis technique. Advocates of the grounded theoretical method also have a curious tendency to rarely venture beyond the concept development stage of research. That is to say, qualitative researchers tend to avoid developing formal hypotheses out of 'grounded' research projects. Perhaps the offshoot of a common tendency to disavow or distrust positivistic research in general, grounded theoreticians are reluctant to progress with the methodological to its logical (and instructed) terminus. Without advancing general, testable theoretical principles from grounded research, qualitative research runs the inevitable risk of being classified as esoteric, non-generalisable and unreliable.

Beyond the Techniques for Knowing: The 'Real Deal'

In the previous section, I discussed many of the technical aspects of conducting a prototypical grounded, realist ethnography. When I lead undergraduate or graduate courses in research methodology, I review those techniques in painstaking detail in order to impress upon students the rigours involved in conducting realist ethnography in the pursuit of theories of culture grounded in the messy, complicated, surprising and sometimes maddening nature of people's daily lives. But curious students always ask more about the method, probing and challenging me to recount the major stumbling blocks or points of frustration in doing ethnography. I am happy to oblige these questions, as this point is where the truth about realist ethnography as a form of social interaction and modality of living for the researcher surfaces.

Ethnographies, in any manifestation, thrive or fizzle out depending on the researcher's ability to gain access (and willingness to access) to the setting or culture of interest. Consider the following example. When I decided to conduct an ethnographic field project on Ashtanga yoga, I knew that there were several studios in Toronto offering Ashtanga-like classes. But knowing a few studios or people who practice, then participating in a few classes across the city, is not an entrée into yogic culture. I needed to access and interact with people who lived, breathed and promoted the tradition. I needed to do what they do, see the practice as they see it and understand how their culture makes sense to them as its core enthusiasts. Participating daily at the studio did not secure true entrée either. Only through a willingness to *socialise* with members and live the physical culture provides access. Ethnographers unable or unwilling to access the system of shared meaning and problem solving that is the 'culture' of their interest are faced with a considerable barrier in the knowledge acquisition process.

Access to the core networks of lifestyle participants in a physical culture is only the beginning. Several weeks or months may pass before one secures a role in the group. A basic sociological lesson instructs us that membership in a culture is framed by one's roles, statuses and identities in the group. Why is this important in realist ethnography? Because one actually becomes what we call the 'instrument of data collection' (i.e. you are actually the *recorder* of data every day in the field), how you access the group, what roles you play and how other people position you as a person in the group substantially influence the volume and depth of the information you are able to gather over time. Who you are partially determines what you see, what you are told and what you eventually know. I am fully convinced, for instance, that unless one fully immerses oneself in a culture, say, Ashtanga for example, its members will maintain an arm's length cultural distance from you. As my role took on greater depth and breadth in Ashtanga, the more its culture became 'real' to me on both personal and professional grounds.

Students enthralled with the ethnographic method are often overwhelmed by the open-endedness of the ethnographic task and end up asking, 'what do I collect as data?' Empirical data could be everything and anything one hears, feels, sees, smells and reads in the field. Most of the time, a researcher will only have a vague understanding of what is important at first (i.e. for answering one's initial research question) and so everything is noted, recorded and reflected upon until a dominant theoretical idea or set of main conceptual foci emerge in the study (as discussed in the previous section). Conversations with others, descriptions of interaction, artifacts gathered in the field and places visited need to be recorded in meticulous detail. For example, my interest in retrenchment stirred not from any brilliant quote offered to me in an interview or core passage from the *Yoga Sutras*. I first saw 'retrenchment' one day in morning Mysore practice. Looking around at the bodies moving, I noted how little people wore, the quietness of room, the simple and Spartan nature of the mats and wooden floor, the bleak whiteness of the walls and absence of fancy water bottles, foods or even fans in the room. Interviews with key informants later on in the study provided me with an opportunity to expand my conceptual and substantive curiosities about retrenchment. After interviewing subjects, I also re-read books, magazines and canonical texts to see if my theoretical code had any 'analytical legs' across these data. What generally started as a broad and overwhelming venture into the cultural dark transformed into a defined research venture. Again, there are no magic templates, tricks, tips or steps one may employ in order to develop conceptual clarity in a project.

The topic of objectivity or value-freedom rears its head with clockwork predictability during debates about realist ethnography. My students reactively condemn ethnographic data as 'biased' (a term students 'know' until they are asked to write a working definition of the term), unscientific, coloured by one's personal thoughts and emotions, and therefore totally invalid. I respond with well-worn arguments about the presence of 'subjectivity' in all academic research (i.e. the subjects researchers selectively prefer, the partial questions we ask, favoured theories we explore and methods we chose, and so on), and claim that true scientific objectivity is more of a golem or phantom in research than a reality. But I now also describe how, in the study of Ashtanga, I learned that methodological objectivity may simply mean persistent, single-focused commitment to investigating a culture under study. Stated in another way, objectivity refers to a 'non-attached' devotion to knowing ethnographic others in both idiographic and nomothetic ways. I came to realise that what Elias (1987) describes, in methodological terms, as 'involved detachment' as a technique of/for knowing sociological truths is the conceptual cousin to the pursuit of vairagya through abhyasa in the world of Ashtanga yoga.

And then, of course, we traverse among the most difficult subjects: how to write and represent culture through a text. Contemporary journal articles in the SPC field which often purport to be ethnographic scarcely read or feel ethnographic at all. As Newman and Giardina (2011) describe, SPC ethnographic articles are often overly sterile, disembodied and atheoretical tomes. Voices from the field disappear, 'thick descriptions' and ideas stemming from field notes or observations are absent and richly layered representations of social scenes, settings and encounters 'out there' are forsaken. But sociological (ethnographic) accounts of the world are most compelling when they are theoretically generative, yes, but also descriptively rich, colourful and conversational with a reader. Among the most valuable insights provided by the contemporary ethnographic modes of knowing like mobile, visual, photo, sensory and queer methods (as showcased in this book) is the idea that transforming complex, dynamic and into an inter-actively flat or 'dead' academic text ranks as the worst of sins committed by the modern qualitative researcher.

The discussion of research ethics proves to be one of the liveliest around the subject of (realist) ethnography. Van den Hoonaard (2003) rightfully suggests that the moral panic regarding the litany of 'ethical dilemmas' in the field has persuaded research ethics boards (REBs) across universities to grow increasingly sceptical about ethnography in general. Without question, several of my studies (like that of ticket scalping in particular) would likely face a stern rejection from my own REB at the University of Toronto today. The study of Ashtanga, though, posed few of the traditional ethnographic worries (safety, power differentials, vulnerability of participants and inability to consent) for REB members and others. Akin to Sugden's argument in Chapter 11, I advocate a full disclosure of my research role, interests, observational practices and desire for interviews with subjects as social 'grease' facilitating the process of membership in a group. I have found, quite consistently across incredibly varied social groups, that people like Ashtangis loved being studied in most cases; they love being questioned and being the star of a study. Knowing that an academic finds good enough cause to examine something one is interested in provides a certain amount of cultural capital and social bragging rights to group members.

With the above said, one never fully discloses one's personal (let alone academic) thoughts, feelings and interpretations of the group being studied. The failure to disclose one's thoughts is tantamount to lying; at least from a narrowly framed REB perspective. But from another, it strategically mimics the sort of 'lying' we do with/to people in the normal course of cultural life; as such it is part of being situated in a group like Ashtangis. I never discussed, for example, my critical thoughts about certain practitioners' apparent interests only in asanas and not the other limbs of the practice, or contradictions posed by some practitioners' lifestyles of consumption and faith in yoga. At times, I met particular people in the group who I found abrasive, believed were liars, and I felt like confronting them at times. Humans interact in the field, not robots, and these scenarios naturally arise. Remaining silent may be preferred in one instance – not as a matter of protecting the 'vulnerable' from being upset, but because vocalising one's opinions so might close interactive doors. But at other times, as Andy Hathaway and I (Hathaway & Atkinson, 2003) described, confronting or challenging people in the field (and in some ways making them deliberately uncomfortable) about their statements or activities is a vital tool of data collection and may pave the way for considerable learning – again, these confrontations occur as a natural part of human group life.

Finally, no research ethics manual or textbook to date (at least those I have perused) instructs as to how friendships are to be managed in the field. I have developed wonderful friendships through the ethnographic act on Ashtanga, and I believe the scientific, substantive and socially evocative qualities of ethnographic texts are ultimately reflections of the breadth and depth of friendships cultivated in the field. Truly befriending others is the ethnographic method. I started to learn the most about Ashtanga when I stopped seeing other practitioners in the shala as subjects doing the practice, and when I had grown to know them as friends in a mutually constituted community involved in Ashtanga. The path to intersubjectivity and the co-production of cultural/ethnographic knowledge is achieved when one is physically, emotionally and socially emplaced in a community, but still has a critical sensitivity to the sociological task at hand. The most important ethical principle of realist ethnography I know is to allow culture to be written on you as much as you will, in turn, eventually seize the mandate to write culture.

REALIST CONTROVERSIES

The belief that ethnographic accounts can be 'realist' (i.e. textually represent the complexities of social life in an accurate manner) has come under consistent scrutiny for over forty years (Clough, 1992; Hammersley, 1992). In the first instance, fervent advocates of more 'scientific'/positivistic methods of data collection question the reliability (repeatability) and external validity of realist ethnographic findings. In the second instance, influential qualitative methodologists like Norman Denzin (2003) have convinced scores of contemporary ethnographers to abandon the pursuit of metaphysical realism in their qualitative efforts. Today, the methodological zeitgeist in qualitative academic circles promotes research on the hyper-construction of social life; it promulgates an ontological position that portrays human actors as entirely too fragmented, radically contextual and 'intersectional' to be understood through realist tales.

Both traditional positivists and the growing legions of neo-ethnographers question the empirical value of pursuing generalised ethnographic truths. With different methodological foci and emphases, they might ask, could another person have studied Ashtanga in Toronto and compiled the very same (or at least similar) story of the setting as me? Probably not, because ethnography relies upon, and is produced through, the intermixing of roles, relationships and personalities in the field. As a related concern, can a realist ethnographer ever represent the reality of everyday cultural life in an accurate manner? Can the stories I write about Ashtanga be convincingly told as a generalisable depiction of cultural membership and experience? Is there even such thing as 'an' Ashtanga culture and is there 'a' member?

Realist ethnographies suffer from a fermenting belief among qualitative researchers that any academic attempt to portray a culture and its members academically (in a reduced, generalised story about said culture) is partly an act of academic thievery (Van Maanen, 2001). Voices, critics tell us, are often 'stolen' from the field without compensation, assembled to suit the researcher's theoretical purposes and disfigured into inaccessible, verbose academic speak. Realist ethnographic research is viewed as an act of cultural colonialism the privileges the powerful researcher as the author(ity) of other people's cultures (Reinharz, 1992). This methodological tack shows considerable connections to pervasive theorising in SPC studies about hyper-individualism, ideological implosion in the West, identity-rights movements and associated politics, and the degree to which scholars in the field (and rightfully so) have called into question how minority groups have been systematically excluded from the historical creation of knowledge about SPC. From these perspectives, methodological preference must be given to allowing people to speak for themselves through innovative textual means; to eschewing the notion of universal or generic cultural truths (because the promotion of this scientific construct has been lobbied for by relatively homogeneous white, male, middle-class scholars); to abdicating one's proclaimed role as a decoder of culture; to performing hyper-reflexivity about the nature of one's 'position' (identities) in the research process; to apologising for potentially generalising from the data and, for attempting to represent living, moving cultural processes through standard textual means. These notions have mimetically distributed throughout the sociology of SPC for nearly two decades now, without any sustained (or concatenated) critical analysis or response from methodological experts in the area (Atkinson, 2011; Silk & Andrews, 2011).

My own foray into the world of Ashtanga yoga instructs (at least to me) that realism is not only possible, it is alive and well in the cultures we study (when we choose to study them empirically). Quite simply, cultural values are shared, social experiences are common and salient across diverse people, realities are configured and enacted upon with striking patterns and regularity, and cultural and existential truths are experienced as 'obdurate' in many ways. When attending to the common fears, wishes, angers, experiences, desires and constructions of life expressed and performed by people 'out there' in the field, we learn a great deal about the common experiential tissues binding us together into cultures. These can be, I feel, observed, discussed, dissected, checked, probed, known and ultimately represented by the realist ethnographer. To be sure, people's lives are strikingly similar when we allow our minds to see the similarities, and the fragmented, lonely, anomic nature of hyper reality so often described by late modern qualitative researchers may be more of a product of late modern social philosophy than any empirical reality.

FIVE KEY READINGS

1. Clough, P. (1992). *The end(s) of ethnography: From realism to social criticism.* **London: Sage.**
Clough's text provides a critical analysis of the rise of realist ontologies and epistemologies in the social sciences, and their fall from grace during the 1980s. It is a poignant and predictive text, outlining the major dilemmas facing those who believe in ethnographic metaphysics.

2. Denzin, N. (2003). *Performance ethnography: Critical pedagogy and the politics of culture.* **Thousand Oaks, CA: Sage.**
Denzin's book ushered in a new generational sensibility regarding the why's, what's and how's of ethnography and ethnographic representation. The book is as much a call for a new philosophy of knowing as it is a call to 'think differently' about the purpose of academic research.

3. Elias, N. (1987). *Involvement and detachment.* **Oxford, UK: Basil Blackwell.**
Elias' book is now regarded as a classic statement on sociological method. It explores how people orient themselves in their world, by means of ideals, fantasy beliefs, wishful thinking, fact-related knowledge or feeling impulses, such as hope and fear.

48   MICHAEL ATKINSON

4. Prus, R. (1996). *Symbolic interaction and ethnographic research: Inter-subjectivity and the study of human lived experience.* **Albany, UK: Suny Press.**
This book, by a leading interactionist theorist and methodologist in North America, provides a historical account of the ethnographic method in sociology/social sciences. Prus defends the notion of realism in ethnographic research, and outlines generic processed of human group life to which ethnographers should be attentive.

5. Van Maanen, J. (2001). *Tales from the field: On writing ethnography,* **(2nd ed.). Chicago, IL: University of Chicago Press.**
This is a book about the practice of 'fieldwork' and the various ways culture is written through ethnography. In particular, van Maanen outlines three forms or genres of cultural representation through ethnography – realist tales, confessional tales and impressionist tales. He further raises issues concerning authorial voice, style, truth, objectivity and point of view in ethnography.

REFERENCES

Alexander, B. (2005). Performance ethnography: The re-enacting and inciting of culture. In N. Denzin & Y. Lincoln (Eds.), *Handbook of qualitative inquiry* (3rd ed., pp. 411–441). Thousand Oaks, CA: Sage.
Atkinson, M. (2000). Brother, can you spare a seat: Developing recipes of knowledge in the ticket scalping subculture. *Sociology of Sport Journal, 17,* 151–170.
Atkinson, M. (2011). *Key concepts in sport, exercise and health research methods.* London: Sage.
Atkinson, M., & Young, K. (2008). *Deviance and social control in sport.* Champaign, IL: Human Kinetics.
Beal, B. (1995). Disqualifying the official: An exploration of social resistance through the subculture of skateboarding. *Sociology of Sport Journal, 12,* 226–252.
Charmaz, K. (2003). *Constructing grounded theory: A practical guide through grounded analysis.* London: Sage.
Clough, P. (1992). *The end(s) of ethnography: From realism to social criticism.* London: Sage.
Darnell, S. (2010). Sport, race and bio-politics: Encounters with difference in 'sport for development and peace' internships. *Journal of Sport and Social Issues, 34,* 396–417.
de Garis, L. (1999). Experiments in pro wrestling: Toward a performative and sensuous sport ethnography. *Sociology of Sport Journal, 16,* 65–67.
Denzin, N. (2003). *Performance ethnography: Critical pedagogy and the politics of culture.* Thousand Oaks, CA: Sage.
Elias, N. (1987). *Involvement and detachment.* Oxford, UK: Basil Blackwell.
Finley, S. (2005). Arts-based inquiry: Performing revolutionary pedagogy. In N. Denzin & Y. Lincoln (Eds.), *Handbook of qualitative inquiry* (3rd ed., pp. 681–694). Thousand Oaks, CA: Sage.
Geertz, C. (1973). *The interpretation of cultures.* New York: Basic Books.
Glaser, B. (2001). *The grounded theory perspective: News conceptualisation contrasted with description.* Mill Valley: Sociology Press.

Gold, R. (1958). Roles in sociological field observation. *Social Forces, 36*, 213–217.

Gubrium, J., & Holstein, J. (1997). *The new language of qualitative method.* New York: Oxford University Press.

Hammersley, M. (1992). *What's wrong with ethnography? Methodological explorations.* London: Routledge.

Hathaway, A., & Atkinson, M. (2003). Active interview tactics in research on public deviance: Exploring the two cop personas. *Field Methods, 15*, 161–185.

Hockey, J. (2006). Sensing the run: Distance running and the senses. *The Senses and Society, 1*, 183–202.

Howe, P. (2001). An ethnography of pain and injury in professional rugby union: The case of Pontypridd RFC. *International Review for the Sociology of Sport, 36*(3), 289–303.

Kemmis, S., & McTaggart, R. (2005). Participatory action research: Communicative action and the public sphere. In N. Denzin & Y. Lincoln (Eds.), *Handbook of qualitative inquiry* (3rd ed., pp. 559–603). Thousand Oaks, CA: Sage.

Monaghan, L. (2001). *Bodybuilding, drugs and risk.* London: Routledge.

Newman, J., & Giardina, M. (2011). *Sport, spectacle and NASCAR nation.* London: Palgrave Macmillan.

Pink, S. (2009). *Doing visual ethnography.* London: Sage.

Prus, R. (1996). *Symbolic interaction and ethnographic research: Intersubjectivity and the study of human lived experience.* Albany, NY: Suny Press.

Reinharz, S. (1992). *Feminist methods in social research.* Oxford, UK: Oxford University Press.

Sands, R. (2001). *Sport ethnography.* Champaign, IL: Human Kinetics.

Silk, M. (2001). The conditions of practice: Television production practices at Kuala Lumpur 98. *Sociology of Sport Journal, 18*, 277–301.

Silk, M., & Andrews, D. (2011). Toward a physical cultural studies. *Sociology of Sport Journal, 28*, 4–35.

Smith, D. (1987). *The everyday world as problematic: A feminist sociology.* Boston, MA: Northeastern University Press.

Strauss, A., & Corbin, J. (1998). *Basics of qualitative research: Grounded theory, procedures and techniques.* Newbury Park, CA: Sage.

Thorpe, H. (2011). *Snowboarding bodies in theory and practice.* London: Palgrave.

Van den Hoonaard, W. (2003). *Walking the tightrope: Ethical issues for qualitative researchers.* Toronto: University of Toronto Press.

Van Maanen, J. (2001). *Tales from the field: On writing ethnography* (2nd ed.). Chicago, IL: University of Chicago Press.

Wacquant, L. (2004). *Body and soul: Ethnographic notebooks of an apprentice-boxer.* New York: Oxford University Press.

Wheaton, B. (2000). 'Just do it': Consumption, commitment, and identity in the windsurfing subculture. *Sociology of Sport Journal, 17*, 254–274.

Williams, R. (1977). *Marxism and literature.* Oxford, UK: University of Oxford Press.

Willis, P. (1998). Theoretical confessions and reflexive method. In K. Gelder & S. Thornton (Eds.), *The subcultures reader* (pp. 246–251). New York: Routledge.

Wilson, B., & Atkinson, M. (2005). Rave and straightedge, the virtual and the real: Exploring online and offline experiences in Canadian youth subcultures. *Youth & Society, 36*, 276–311.

Wilson, B., & Sparks, B. (1996). It's gotta be the shoes: Youth, race, and sneaker commercials. *Sociology of Sport Journal, 13*, 398–427.

Wolcott, H. (1999). *Ethnography: A way of seeing.* New York: Altamira.

CHAPTER 3

THE ETHNOGRAPHIC (I)NTERVIEW IN THE SPORTS FIELD: TOWARDS A POSTMODERN SENSIBILITY

Holly Thorpe

ABSTRACT

Purpose – *The purpose of the chapter is to introduce interviewing as an exploratory research approach for understanding the lived experiences of individuals and groups in sports and physical cultural contexts. The author draws on her own research with snowboarders to illustrate some of the standard and unique issues related to conducting interviews as part of ethnographic fieldwork.*

Design/methodology/approach – *The chapter begins with a brief history of the development of qualitative interviews and their various uses in sport studies. The author then provides a description of her use of 'postmodern-inspired' interviews as part of a broader ethnographic study of snowboarding culture. Following this, she adopts an alternative representational approach to illustrate some of the practical, ethical, political and embodied issues for reflexive researchers working in the critical paradigm and conducting interviews in sport and physical cultural fields.*

Qualitative Research on Sport and Physical Culture
Research in the Sociology of Sport, Volume 6, 51–78
Copyright © 2012 by Emerald Group Publishing Limited
All rights of reproduction in any form reserved
ISSN: 1476-2854/doi:10.1108/S1476-2854(2012)0000006006

Findings – *The chapter illustrates the value of a postmodern approach to interviewing that recognises the interview as more than textual, and gives greater consideration to the affective, sensuous, relational, embodied and socio-spatial dimensions of each interview event.*

Research limitations/implications – *The chapter examines the strengths and limitations of qualitative interviewing, with particular attention to the potential and perils of interviewing in the sports field.*

Originality/value – *The chapter provides a succinct introduction to the use of interviewing in sport and physical culture, and makes an innovative contribution by focusing on ethnographic interviews.*

Keywords: Interviews; semi-structured; ethnography; fieldwork; reflexivity; snowboarding

INTRODUCTION

Whether it is the cover story for the latest issue of *Sports Illustrated*, a documentary about big wave surfing, a televised post-game debrief with the captain of a champion basketball team or a *CNN* investigative feature into coach–athlete relationships, interviews are central to the production and consumption of contemporary sport and physical culture (SPC). The ubiquity and significance of interviews in sport today is perhaps not surprising given that Westerners are, according to Silverman (1997), living in 'interview societies' (p. 248). The interview – seen in various forms of news items, talk shows, documentaries and job applications – "pervades and produces our contemporary cultural experiences and knowledges of authentic personal, private selves" (Rapley, 2004, p. 15) in various social spheres, including SPC.

The interview is also a central method in critical research on SPC. Scholars are engaging a panorama of techniques including (but not limited to) formal, semi-structured, unstructured, face-to-face, electronic, individual interviews, focus groups and oral histories, to gain fresh insights into the lived experiences of individuals and groups in various sporting contexts. In this chapter, I focus on one type of interviewing that, despite being popular among critical SPC researchers, has gained relatively little detailed scholarly attention. Here, I am referring to conducting interviews as part of broader ethnographic projects. Most books focusing on qualitative research methods feature separate chapters on fieldwork and interviews (e.g. Andrews, Mason, & Silk, 2005; Denzin & Lincoln, 2011; Markula & Silk, 2011; c.f. Atkinson & Coffey, 2003; Sherman Heyl, 2002). But, for many scholars, conducting ethnographic studies of SPCs, interviews are an integral part of fieldwork. Thus, in this chapter, I examine the potential and perils of doing reflexive, embodied and ethical interviews in the fields of SPC. Drawing upon examples from my ethnographic research on snowboarding culture, I examine some of the distinctive practical, political, ethical and embodied characteristics of interviewing in sport and physical cultural environments. In so doing, I argue that interviewing in fields of SPCs requires a dynamic, flexible, relational, reflexive and theoretically informed approach, or what might be called a postmodern approach. With examples from my own research experiences, I also advocate the need to recognise the interview as more than textual, and to give greater consideration to the affective, sensuous, embodied and socio-spatial dimensions of each interview event.

THE QUALITATIVE INTERVIEW: A BRIEF HISTORY

Interviews are a central method within the social sciences, with some estimating that they are involved in up to 90 per cent of social science investigations (Holstein & Gubrium, 2003). Yet, the popularity of the qualitative interview is a relatively recent development (Platt, 2002). The first social survey has been attributed to Charles Booth who, in 1886, used surveys in conjunction with unstructured interviews and ethnographic observations, to conduct a comprehensive study of the economic and social conditions of the people of London. Similar approaches were adopted in studies of various cities in England and America during the late nineteenth and early twentieth centuries. It was not until World War II, however, that the standardised survey interview was used to garner broader 'public opinion' on an array of social issues ranging from women's lingerie collections to education to 'attitudes towards coloured people' (de Castella, 2011, para. 5). Following the War, quantitative survey research became 'the method of choice' in sociology (Fontana & Frey, 2000, p. 648). Quantitative interviews dominated the field for the next three decades, although qualitative interviews were increasingly used during the 1970s, 1980s and 1990s, often hand in hand with ethnographic methods such as participant observation.

Many of the early studies employing qualitative interviews assumed some of the 'quantifiable scientific rigor that so preoccupied survey research'

(Fontana & Frey, 2000, p. 649). According to Oakley (1981), textbook advice on interviewing during this period confirmed:

(a) its status as a mechanical instrument of data-collection; (b) its function as a specialised form of conversation in which one person asks the questions and another gives the answers; (c) its characterization of interviewees as essentially passive individuals, and (d) its reduction of interviewers to a question asking and rapport-promoting role. (p. 36)

The qualitative interview was, however, 'revolutionised' in the late 1970s and 1980s (Holstein & Gubrium, 2003, p. 4) during the general 'interpretivist' turn in Europe and North America that recognised the limitations of positivism, and particularly the dominance of grand narratives and assumptions of objectivity and truth, for understanding the complexities and nuances of individuals lived experiences within particular social settings (Denzin, 1978). Such epistemological debates in the social sciences and humanities, and particularly concerns expressed by feminist and postmodern ethnographers, challenged assumptions underpinning formal, structured interviews (Holstein & Gubrium, 2003). Of particular concern was the relationship between the researcher and their 'subject', which some scholars argued was unethical. More specifically, building upon Oakley's (1981) foundational critiques of the power dimensions underlying the interview exchange, Fontana and Frey (1994) proclaimed, 'the techniques and tactics of interviewing are really ways of manipulating respondents while treating them as objects or numbers rather than individual human beings' (p. 373). Feminist scholars were instrumental in prompting interviewers to move beyond 'universalist positions in moral philosophy (duty ethics of principles, utilitarian ethics of consequences)' and to 'recognise relationships with research participants as an ethical issue' (Olesen, 2011, p. 136). In advocating the need for greater sensitivity to 'relational ethics' and issues of power, agency, authority, reflexivity and representation, feminist and postmodern ethnographers helped transform the way researchers were 'thinking about and using interviews and their data' (Holstein & Gubrium, 2003, p. 4).

Formal, structured interviews continue to be employed by scholars in an array of fields, including education, psychology and sociology. But, for those working in the interpretivist paradigm, the qualitative interview has been re-imagined as 'inherently interactional, reflexive and intersubjective' (Sin, 2003, p. 305). As Holstein and Gubrium (2003) proclaim, the qualitative interview should be conceptualised as a context-specific 'social encounter in which knowledge is constructed' in dialogue with participants, rather than a 'simple information-gathering operation' (p. 4). In his examination of this divide in interviewing philosophies, Seale (1998) identifies two major traditions, 'interview-data-as-resource' and 'interview-data-as-topic'. In the former, interview data collected are seen as '(more or less) reflecting the interviewees' reality outside the interview', whereas in the interview-data-as-topic approach, interview data are seen as '(more or less) reflecting a reality jointly constructed by the interviewee and interviewer' (cited in Rapley, 2001, p. 303). Working within the latter, Rapley (2001) describes interview 'data' as always highly dependent on, and emerging from, 'the specific local interactional context which is produced in and through the talk (and concomitant identity work) of the interviewee *and the interviewer*' (p. 303; italics in original).

Others refer to a postmodern approach to interviewing that privileges 'the conversational, the narrative, the linguistic, the contextual and the inter-relational nature of knowledge' (Kvale, 2007, p. 21; also see Alversson, 2002; Fontana, 2002; Fontana & Prokos, 2007; Roulston, 2010). Building upon and extending this approach, some are engaging alternative modes of representing data generated from interviews to engage audiences 'in new ways, often outside the academy' (Roulston, 2010, p. 219). For example, rather than viewing the interview as a 'method for gathering information', Denzin (2001) has conceptualised the 'reflexive, dialogic, or performative interview' as 'a vehicle for producing performance texts and performance ethnographies about self and society' (p. 24). For Denzin (2001), the aim of the performative interview is to 'bring people together' and 'criticise the world the way it is, and offer suggestions about how it could be different' (p. 24).

Today, the positions adopted by qualitative researchers vary considerably with much debate as to what are the most ethical and effective relationships between interviewers and their research participants, and understandings of interview data as offering access to either 'true' knowledge or partial and situated accounts of individuals and groups lived experiences. The potential for alternative representations of knowledge generated via interviews to create broader political and social change is also hotly contested. There is, however, 'broad-based commitment' among those working in interpretivist traditions to conduct interviews ethically, that is, for researchers to show due respect and avoid harming in anyway those who willingly share their time, opinions, memories and experiences for the purposes of research (Sherman Heyl, 2002, p. 370). Laurel Richardson (1992) calls this commitment 'relational ethics' and it involves 'honouring and empowering' those 'who teach me about their lives ... even if they and I see their worlds differently' (p. 108).

[handwritten annotation: assumptions, ideals & ideas for research, can end up informing their entire research]

Qualitative interviews are used extensively in sociological and, to a lesser extent, psychological and historical research on sport, exercise and physical culture. Although individualistic semi-structured face-to-face interviews are the most common form of interview in critical sport studies, other interviewing styles (e.g. focus groups, oral history, unstructured, electronic) are also being used to understand the experiences, memories and inter-pretations of individuals and groups within various sporting contexts. Different ontological and epistemological assumptions underpin these various approaches and influence the 'many how-to-do decisions through-out an interview investigation' (Kvale, 2007, p. 22), including the parti-cipants selected, design of interview guide, relationship between interviewer and interviewee, data analysis and presentation, and the use of theory (Markula & Silk, 2011).

While some researchers discuss and debate the merit of different interview styles – for example semi-structured versus unstructured, face-to-face versus electronic, individual versus group – Roulston (2010) offers a valuable contribution to these debates by identifying broader thematic tendencies in methodological literature on qualitative interviews. She offers a six-fold typology of interviewing. She labels her categories neo-positivist, romantic, constructionist, postmodern, transformative and decolonising. In so doing, Roulston (2010) makes explicit the important point that researchers' theoretical assumptions about qualitative interviews have 'implications for how research interviews are structured, the kinds of questions made possible, the kinds of interview questions posed, how data might be analysed and represented, how research projects are designed and conducted, and how the quality of the research is judged by the communities of practice in which work is situated' (p. 224). Like Roulston, I too have seen many emerging researchers confidently conclude their data-gathering process only to embark on a desperate bid to find the theory that 'neatly … fits the data' (Baert, 2004, p. 367). Arguably, regardless of their theoretical leanings, emerging *and* experienced critical scholars of SPC should begin their projects by carefully considering how their ontological, epistemological, theoretical and political assumptions might (implicitly and explicitly) inform their entire investigation, from developing research questions, selecting participants, designing research guides and relationships with participants to transcription, analysis and the representation of participant voices.

It is beyond the scope of this chapter to provide an overview of the various styles of interviewing popular among sport scholars, and the episte-mological and theoretical assumptions underpinning each approach. Rather, I draw upon examples of my own work with snowboarders to discuss the potential and perils of conducting postmodern-inspired qualitative interviews. The remainder of this chapter consists of two parts. First, I provide a description of my use of interviews as part of a broader ethnographic study of snowboarding culture. Second, I adopt an alternative representational approach to illustrate practical, ethical, political and embodied issues for reflexive researchers working in the critical paradigm and conducting interviews in sport and physical cultural fields.

INTERVIEWING IN THE SPORTS FIELD: AN ETHNOGRAPHIC STUDY OF SNOWBOARDING CULTURE

In my recent book *Snowboarding Bodies in Theory and Practice*, I offer a multidimensional understanding of snowboarding bodies as historical, gendered, represented, cultural, moving, travelling, sensual, affective and political. Working within the critical paradigm, I wanted to identify and explain the multiple forms of power operating on and through snowboarding bodies in historical and contemporary contexts (see Thorpe, 2011). My understanding of the complexities of snowboarding bodies derived from multiple modes of data generation, a type of methodology used extensively by Bourdieu and which he describes as 'discursive montage' of '*all sources*' (Bourdieu & Wacquant, 1992, p. 66, emphasis added). Similarly, Grossberg (2001) recommends using 'any and every kind of empirical method, whatever seems useful to the particular project' in order to 'gather more and better information, descriptions, resources', and improve one's interpretations (cited in Wright, 2001, p. 145). Throughout this project, I seized all types of data, evidence, sources and artefacts to enlighten my inquiry into snowboarding bodies.

According to Mills (1959), sociologists do not study projects; rather, they become tuned, or sensitive, to themes that 'they see and hear everywhere in [their] experience' (p. 211). As I became increasingly sensitive to the themes of the snowboarding body, I gathered evidence from personal observations and experiences, magazines, websites, newspapers, interviews and personal communications, videos, Internet chat rooms, promotional material, television programs, press releases, public documents, reports from snowboarding's administrative bodies and promotional material from sporting organisations and from associated industries. While my use of interviews is the focus of this chapter, it is important to note that I used this method in conjunction with other ethnographic methods, particularly participant observations and media analysis, to help develop a more intimate understanding of the complexities, nuances and contradictions within snowboarding culture.

The ethnographic approach adopted in this study was atypical in that, rather than focusing upon a particular site, I adopted a multi-sited, 'global ethnographic' approach with the aim of examining the values, practices and interactions unique to local snowboarding cultures, as well as regional, national and global flows of people, objects, value systems, information and images within and across these places (Burawoy et al., 2000). Attempting to further expand my understanding of the complexities of snowboarding bodies, I conducted 15 'ethnographic visits' – ranging from one week to one month – in an array of snowboarding communities and ski resorts in Canada, France, Italy, New Zealand, Switzerland and the United States, between 2004 and 2010. Attempting to understand how snowboarders experienced their bodies in (and across) local snowboarding fields, I made observations on and off the snow (including lift lines, chair lifts, resort lodges, snowboard competitions, prize giving events, video premiers, bars, cafes, local hangouts, snowboard shops, bus-shelters, train stations, airports). During this fieldwork, I observed, listened, engaged in analysis and made mental notes, switching from snowboarder to researcher depending on the requirements of the situation (Thorpe, 2011).

During my multiple phases of fieldwork, I conducted semi-structured (and a small number of unstructured) interviews with 60 participants (32 female and 28 male) from an array of countries, including Australia, Canada, England, France, New Zealand, South Africa, Switzerland and the United States. Distinct from casual conversations in the field, interviews were organised for a particular time and place with select individuals who I identified as having the potential to offer fresh insights into particular dimensions of their own and/or others snowboarding bodies. I conducted interviews with snowboarders I met in the field, as well as contacts made prior to, and following, visits to particular locations. Interviewees ranged from 18 to 56 years of age, and included novice snowboarders, recreational snowboarders or 'weekend warriors', committed/core boarders, professional snowboarders, an Olympic snowboarder, an Olympic judge, snowboarding journalists, photographers, film-makers, magazine editors, snowboard company owners, snowboard shop employees and owners, snowboard instructors and coaches, and event organisers and judges. Interviews ranged from 30 minutes to 4 hours, depending on the willingness of participants, and were conducted in an array of locations typically chosen by the interviewee (e.g. café, bar, ski resort restaurant, at a film premier or snowboarding competition). As per the requirements of my university ethics committee, all interviewees received both an information sheet that outlined the project and their ethical rights, and a consent form. All interviewees had the choice to remain anonymous (full confidentiality), to be partially identified (e.g. occupation and/or first name) or to be fully identified (full name and occupation), and signed the consent forms accordingly. While all but two agreed to be fully identified, in my published work all interviewees are given pseudonyms, except where the participant agreed to full disclosure and identifiers (e.g. age, occupation) help contextualise a particular comment or example included in the text.

Snowball Sampling

→ participants tell people they know about study for recruitment.

Magazines, websites and email were invaluable for identifying and making contact with potential interviewees prior to commencing the interview phase of fieldwork. Many of my interviewees, however, were met during phases of participant observation, often via happenchance conversations in various locations in the field (e.g. chairlifts, snowboard shops, in cafes). For example, a conversation with an Australian female snowboard instructor on a chairlift at a resort in Canada led to an interview in a local café later in the day. During the interview, two of the interviewee's friends entered the café and, after introducing me and explaining that I was doing research on snowboarding culture and interested in talking to female snowboarders about their experiences, I had confirmed another two interviews for the following day. As this example suggests, the snowball method of sampling proved effective with many participants helping me gain access to other key informants by offering names, contact details (e.g. email addresses, phone numbers) and even vouching for my authenticity as 'a researcher who actually snowboards' (field notes, November 2005). Importantly, however, the snowball method of sampling requires an opportunistic and dogged approach – various individuals denied my requests for an interview. However, taking careful notes throughout the recruiting process – the successes and the failures, and the reasons people gave for not taking part – provided valuable insights into the snowboarding culture, as well as the interpretations others made of my researcher/snowboarder identity.

Interviewing Style

Adopting a semi-structured interviewing style, I developed a guide with a selection of key themes and questions prior to each interview. The guides were helpful in preparing me for the interview, and I typically spent some time studying the key themes before meeting the participant. As a relatively inexperienced interviewer, I referred to my guide regularly throughout the interview, particularly when interviewing 'intimidating' individuals such as professional athletes. But, as I gained experience and confidence in my interviewing skills, I found myself using the pre-prepared guides less during the interview, opting instead for a more flexible and conversational dialogue in which I adjusted the structure of questions and followed new directions in relation to the interviewee's responses and the nature of our interaction. During the interviews, I asked participants to reflect on their beliefs about various aspects of the snowboarding culture and encouraged them to express their attitudes, ideas, perceptions and memories on different aspects of the snowboarding body (e.g. gender, media, performance, competition, travel, pleasure, risk, injury, consumption and lifestyle). While key themes ran through many of the interviews, each guide was individualised to the participant. Most of my interviews were semi-structured, yet occasionally a spontaneous interview arose in the field in which I was unable to prepare a guide (see narrative below). In these unstructured interviews, however, I often identified common themes which I was able to explore further with prompts and probes learned from past interview experiences.

While conducting both semi-structured and unstructured interviews, I did not remain neutral or passive (read objective). Rather, I aimed to construct an environment where the interview participants' interpretive capabilities were 'activated, stimulated, and cultivated' (Holstein & Gubrium, 1995, cited in Markula & Pringle, 2006, p. 105). Occasionally I attempted to facilitate rapport and prompt discussion by sharing some of my own snowboarding experiences during the interview. This strategy proved particularly valuable during interviews with individuals who I did not know prior to commencing my research. The majority of participants welcomed further communication (e.g. 'If you want me to clarify anything or answer any other questions, just let me know'), and thus most interviews were followed up with further in-person communications or email discussions.

Electronic Communications

To accommodate the nomadic existence of many snowboarders, I also distributed follow-up interviews via email to 35 participants living or travelling abroad. In some cases, the email interview pre-empted the face-to-face interview. For example, the following email from a professional Canadian snowboarder (met many years prior to commencing my research) reveals both the willingness of some snowboarders to engage in electronic communication and the extent of snowball sampling amongst participants themselves:

> April 2008: Hi Holly Dave mentioned he caught up with you in Whistler a few weeks ago. Sorry I missed you, I was at a comp at Mammoth. Dave said you are doing some interesting research and passed on your questionnaire to me, so I took the liberty of filling it out. It seemed a bit lengthy when I started so I was only planning on doing a bit of it, but ended up filling in the whole thing … it was pretty interesting, got me thinking about some things I don't think I've ever actually put into words before. And [it was] much better than spending my day doing actual work. I've done several other similar reviews and interviews on snowboarding, but this one is more realistic and less 'cheesy' than those. So yeah, it's pretty cool. Ok, hope all is rad and maybe I'll cross paths with you soon. Hang tough and make peace. Eric. (edited for clarity by author)

The majority of respondents wrote freely and in colloquial tones, their comfort with this medium perhaps reflective of the time spent on the Internet for emailing and chatting in their everyday lives. But, as the email from Eric above suggests, my cultural and social capital in the snowboarding field (based on my past participation and relationships with snowboarders) facilitated the use of email interviews, which were always used in conjunction with face-to-face interviews and participant observations in the field.

Transcription and Theoretical Analysis

All face-to-face interviews were recorded via Dictaphone. Some researchers employ professional transcribers to annotate their interview recordings. However, I prefer to transcribe my interviews because I believe it helps me to develop an even more intimate relationship with the interview exchange. Transcribing is a very time-intensive process, often taking me approximately three hours for every one hour of interview dialogue. But, listening to the recordings over and over works to embed participants' reflections and stories in my memory and, as such, is an integral part of my analysis. Indeed, I find the voices of some participants continue to 'speak to me' (sometimes supporting, at other times challenging, my theorising or analysis) years after a particular interview was conducted.

Importantly, a researcher's approach to transcription and analysis is always inextricably linked to their specific theoretical interests (Rapley, 2004). According to Markula and Silk (2011), researchers working in the critical paradigm are 'often vague about how they work with their empirical material':

> This is partly due to their subjective epistemology, which does not necessitate detailed verification of the research process to ensure objectivity. There is a much stronger emphasis on understanding individual meaning making within a social, political, historical and economic context. (p. 109)

In so doing, researchers from the critical paradigm are expected to adopt a well-articulated theoretical frame for interpreting the meanings in interviews, and explain how their theoretical lens informed their analysis. Although some researchers follow the techniques of analysis specific to their theoretical orientation (e.g. Foucualt and genealogy), others do not. Moreover, many theoretical approaches do not advocate a particular style of analysis. Thus, Markula and Silk (2011) offer postmodern researchers some suggestions to facilitate the analysis of interview transcripts, including the identification of themes, analysis of themes, intersections with themes, discrepancies with themes, 'new themes' and 'connection with power relations, theory, and previous literature' (p. 109).

Instead of focusing solely on the detailed structuring of individual interview transcripts, I examined the evolving themes traceable across interviews, as well as identifying new themes and incongruities in the data. Integrating this analysis with participant observations and media analysis further enabled me to examine some of the multiple forms of power operating on and through snowboarding bodies in particular contexts. Using cultural sources, such as magazines, films and websites, in conjunction with multiple phases of fieldwork and interviews, certainly helped deepen my understanding of snowboarding's cultural complexities and the multidimensional snowboarding body. In so doing, the focused and repeated study of interview transcripts enabled me to refine and develop the analytical themes that simultaneously emerged during my participant observations and media analysis, as well as produce new areas of inquiry.

Theory played a fundamental role throughout my investigation of snowboarding bodies, and was integral to enhancing my interpretation of my ethnographic evidence. Throughout my project, I privileged neither theory nor empiricism, instead inferring answers from questions I 'put *to* the evidence and not *from* the sources, which cannot speak for themselves" (Munslow, 2006, p. 49). Rather than adopting a grounded theoretical approach, that involves waiting until the conclusion of the data-gathering phase before generating concepts or theories from emergent themes in the interview transcripts, I refined and developed my ethnographic interpretations throughout the research process by engaging the empirical insights in dialogue with a number of critical theoretical approaches, particularly feminisms, and Bourdieusian and Foucauldian theorising (Thorpe, 2011). In so doing, the theoretical concepts helped direct me to particular sources (including potential interviewees) and set out questions, and they also enabled me to organise evidence and shape explanations of snowboarding bodies. In so doing, each of these theories directed me to particular themes in the interview transcripts, depending on the sociological questions being asked. Nonetheless, throughout my research, I continually sought 'negative instances or contradictory cases' from *all* the sources in order to avoid including only those elements of the snowboarding culture that would substantiate my analyses (Mason, 2002, p. 124).

Representing Voice(s)

Another important consideration is how to represent interview data in the final written report. For researchers using a postmodern conception of interviewing, an underlying assumption is that 'representations of findings are always partial, arbitrary, and situated, rather than unitary, final and holistic' (Roulston, 2010, p. 220). With a postmodern sensibility underpinning my work, I engage multiple (and sometimes contradictory) voices of snowboarders in dialogue with theoretical concepts in my research texts. In conjunction with notes from my fieldwork and other cultural sources (e.g. magazines, films, websites), I use extracts from interviews to bring abstract theoretical concepts 'to life' and to 'provide evidence for particular claims', as well as to 'provide color, add interest, and enhance the legitimacy and credibility of the account' (Amis, 2005, p. 131).

Of course, the reflexive researcher also makes a number of important decisions in representing interview data, including whose voices are included (and excluded), what quotes are selected, how many quotes are included, how quotes are attributed, whether interviewer questions are included and how much contextual information is provided (Amis, 2005). During my research, I found some interviewees more reflective of their cultural experiences and better able to articulate themselves. Some of these individuals became key informants throughout my project, and as such, their voices appear more frequently in some of my published work. However, I also try to illustrate the cultural complexities by presenting comments from participants occupying various positions within the highly fragmented snowboarding culture (e.g. novices, weekend warriors, instructors, professional athletes). When appropriate, I also show that participants are not always in agreement, and in some cases, vehemently oppose the opinions of other snowboarders. In so doing, I illustrate that multiple 'knowledges' co-exist within snowboarding culture. To help the reader make meaning of these multiple voices, I try to position selected quotes within both the macro context – that is, the broader socio-cultural–political context – and the micro context in which the statement was made; I comment on the style of communication (e.g. face-to-face or electronic interview, or conversation in the field), as well as the nationality, age, sex, occupation and/or role within snowboarding culture (e.g. professional athlete, journalist, novice). Where necessary, I also mention my relationship with the participant (e.g. long-time friend, ex-fellow competitor). I also clarify whether the selected quote is representative of the attitudes or perspectives expressed by other interviewees and across other sources (e.g. magazines, websites), or an anomaly in my data.

In describing the perspectives and practices of snowboarding culture, I incorporate numerous voices from interviews, as well as participant observations, magazines, videos and websites, alongside various slogans, clichés and common site- or setting-specific terms. In order to respect participants' style of communication, I do not edit quotes from in-person interviews or email interviews, or websites and magazines; the grammar appears in my published work as it did in the original, except where some basic editing is necessary for clarity. It is important to note, however, that the language of snowboarding culture is highly distinctive; snowboarders have their own argot to describe the snowboard experience, as well as equipment and techniques. Thus, in some texts, I have forewarned the reader of the colourful jargon used, but I do not censor the language used by snowboarders to describe their reflections and experiences in snowboarding culture.

THE ETHNOGRAPHIC (I)NTERVIEW: SOME REFLECTIONS FROM THE FIELD

In the remainder of this chapter, I illustrate some of the procedural messiness of doing interviews in the sports field, and the importance of adopting a dynamic and flexible approach throughout the interview investigation. Inspired by the innovative work of Ellis and Berger (2002), and in an effort 'to move further toward reflexivity, polyvocality, and contextuality' (Markula & Silk, 2011, p. 181), I offer a narrative of an ethnographic interview experience in the larger column on the left below. In the smaller column on the right, I highlight some key issues raised in this narrative, particularly relating to interviews as interactional, inter-subjective, situated, sensual and affective experiences. Readers are encouraged to begin with the left column. I conclude with some thoughts on the importance of adopting a reflexive and embodied approach throughout the interview process.

5:05 pm Thursday, February 2009: Sitting on a bench at the base of a ski resort deep in the Colorado Rockies, my feet ache, my thighs are heavy with fatigue and my right shoulder throbs from a fall in the terrain park around mid-afternoon. The skin on my face is hot, raw and tight. As I wait for my interviewee to arrive, I watch the final skiers and snowboarders sliding down the mountain, unbuckling their bindings and shaking out their legs.

Jeremy – the 'park groomer' – arrives on time and introduces himself briefly before leading me to his 'cat'. Standing on the metal teethed treads, he reaches and opens the door. A little tentatively, I climb up and into the cab. I am surprised by the plush interior, and only have time to note a stack of CDs and a crumpled bag of chips before the beast roars into life. As we plough over the crusted snow, vibrations ripple through my chest cavity and I lose my train of thought.

Picking up his radio, Jeremy chats briefly to other drivers spread across the mountain – I catch snippets of

Preparation for entering the field – prior contact: Prior to my visit, I conducted extensive electronic research on the physical and socio-cultural geography, as well as some of the key snowboarding-related businesses and organisations in the region. This research helped me identify some key themes for investigation, and initiated the snowball sampling process. Initial contact was made via email with the terrain park manager, which I followed up with a text message shortly upon arriving in the ski town.

Interviews in the (snow) field: To make the most of short phases of fieldwork, my days in the field are typically filled with participant observations and interviews. In this instance, I was still information about locations, tasks, times and snow conditions. I note snowboarding stickers on the dashboard, and a cut out picture of a model in a bikini taped to inside of his sun-visor. For a brief moment I feel uncomfortable and nervous about the interview. But, with Jeremy focused on shifting gears, moving levers and scraping the icy face off the quarter-pipe, I remind myself that I am here to do a job too. I take a breath to focus and help myself get into 'character', transitioning from fellow snowboarder to interviewer.

'So, Sam [head of park crew] said he passed on the information sheet about my research. Do you have any questions about my project, or any problem with me recording our discussion so I can remember what we discussed when I get home to New Zealand?' 'Na, no worries. I read the info sheet thingee and somewhere here is the signed formed', he says, digging through a pile of papers on the seat between us, only momentarily taking his eyes off the towering wall of snow on our left. 'Great, so I will just switch on the recorder here. Let me know if you want me to switch it off at anytime, and please just tell me if you don't want to answer a particular question or you would like to end the interview. Also, I should just reinforce that there are no right or wrong answers to my questions. I'm mostly just interested in hearing about your experiences as a terrain park

wearing my snowboarding attire, including soggy snowboard boots and wet gloves. While not particularly conducive for a comfortable interview, my physically active snowboarding body sometimes helped me gain rapport with interviewees.

Ethics and signed consent on site: While conducting fieldwork I always carried information sheets, consent forms and a stack of business cards with a local contact number, in the large pockets of my snowboard pants or jacket. Discussing the ethical details, signing the consent form and introducing the Dictaphone can sometimes disrupt the flow of the dialogue and cause some unease for the interviewee. However, in most cases, this can be covered quickly and effectively, particularly if the participant has already read the information sheet.

Interviews in physical cultural spaces: Due to the busy lives of many committed snowboarders during the winter season, groomer'. 'Yep, I read all that in the forms. So, yeah, just fire away'. Jeremy seems undaunted by the interview situation, and eager to get on with the conversation.

'Ok, great. Well, perhaps you might start by telling me how you got into snowboarding, and then into grooming'. For the next 45 minutes, Jeremy speaks candidly about his life as a snowboarder, and his career as a 'parkie' and then a 'groomer', all the while working systematically through the terrain park digging, and shaping take-offs and landings. Jeremy has strong opinions and offers vivid and emotive responses to my questions. Trying not to break the flow, I glance briefly down at my interview guide. Noting that we have already covered most of my key questions, I begin to wonder what I should ask next. As if on cue, we are blinded by the lights of another groomer heading in our direction. Jeremy tells me he has been summoned to another job on the other side of the mountain, so I need to change vehicles. I thank Jeremy for his time and promise to be in touch shortly via email with his transcript and perhaps a few follow-up questions. 'Yep, no worries, maybe catch ya in the park tomorrow', he yells, as I begin climbing out into the darkness and up into the second machine.

Opening the door, I am surprised to see a petite young woman, no more

some interviews occurred at their place of work (e.g. snowboard shop, ski resort office, inside a snow groomer). Some of these locations are not always ideal for interviewing (e.g. due to background noise, interviewees multitasking, interruptions such as phone calls), but the space, and the interviewee's interactions within it, can also provide valuable cultural knowledge. According to Sin (2003), while the *in situ* nature of interviewing is often overlooked in qualitative research, an interview site can 'reflect or refract the wider social geographies of respondents' and 'yield important information regarding the way respondents construct their identities' (p. 306). This was certainly true of all my interviews conducted in the snow field.

Building rapport: As Henderson (1991) and others have pointed out 'establishing reciprocity, generosity, and responsibility are crucial to the ongoing development of a research relationship' than 20 years old, with long dark hair falling straight from her beanie, sitting behind the controls. I note the label of her beanie and the glint of her studded belt. Before I get a chance to introduce myself, she pushes her boot down on the accelerator and we start climbing up the backside of a jump; the cabin is on a steep angle and gravity forces me into the back of my chair. Calm and in control, she lowers the bucket at the front of the groomer, tearing apart and then flattening the landing.

The young woman's name is Sandra, and I immediately sense her apprehension. After our initial introductions, she asks about my research, when I arrived in town, how long I'm here for, and why I was interviewing Jeremy. I tell her I'm a sociologist at a university in New Zealand and I've spent the past five years researching and writing about snowboarding culture. 'I'm trying to understand snowboarders experiences both on and off the snow in different places around the world. I'm trying to capture the voices and stories from lots of different people involved in snowboarding as a sport, career and lifestyle', I explain. She nods but remains unconvinced.

Attempting to open up the conversation, I note that this is actually the first time in all of my travels that I have seen a young woman driving a groomer, and I ask

(cited in Amis, 2005, p. 120).

Many snow boarders are critical of 'outsiders' infiltrating their culture for commercial or research purposes. Many snow boarders are critical of 'outsiders' infiltrating their culture for commercial or research purposes. Due to the spontaneity of my meeting with Sandra, we were both unprepared for the interaction.. Sandra knew nothing of my research, and she wanted to know who I was, why I was here, and whether I could be trusted. I recognised the need to provide an accessible, informative and honest overview of my past and present research, and to convince Sandra that I was someone worthy of her trust. I felt slightly anxious when Sandra turned the questioning on me. However, Turkel's (1995) comments are encouraging in such moments: 'In the one-to-one interview you start level in the unconfidence, in not knowing where you are going. ... You do it your own way. You experiment. You try this, you try that.

whether she would be willing to tell me about her experiences as a groomer driver. I pull out an information sheet and informed consent form from my pocket. She glances briefly at the pages, before shifting gears and pulling at a leaver that tilts the grate at the front of the groomer. The snow churns beneath us, and I have to tighten my abdominals to minimise the swaying. It's obvious to both of us that she is unable to read these forms right now, so I begin to briefly talk through the information on the sheets. I admit that I am giving her the abbreviated version, but encourage her to read these carefully tomorrow and get back to me with any questions or concerns. 'Okay', her long hair swaying as she nods her head, 'why not'.

Our conversation begins slowly. I tell her about my 'past life' as a competitive snowboarder in New Zealand and an instructor in the United States. We then proceed to share experiences of being women working in the male-dominated ski industry, occasionally laughing at the similarity of some of our anecdotes. I ask whether she has experienced any difficulties as a female groomer driver, and she openly describes her daily frustrations. We have been talking for about 30 minutes when she confides, 'it's so nice to have someone in the cabin that I can talk to. It can get so lonely up here at night. It's not often I get to talk to other women about these

... Stay loose, stay flexible' (cited in Rapley, 2004, p. 30).

Interactional interviewing: As Kvale (2007) so eloquently puts it: 'The knowledge produced depends on the social relationship of interviewer and interviewee, which again rests on the interviewer's ability to create a stage where the subject is free and safe to talk of private events for later public use. This again requires a delicate balance between the interviewer's concern of pursuing interesting knowledge and ethical respect for the integrity of the interview subject' (p. 8).

During interviews, I often shared some of my own experiences with participants to facilitate dialogue and build rapport. According to Oakley (2003), 'when a feminist interviews women ... it becomes clear that, in most cases, the goal of finding out about people through interviewing is best achieved when the relationship between the sorts of things, it's actually really nice'. As the conversation continues, I sense there is something missing from Sandra's story. I probe a little deeper. 'So, how did you get into grooming?'

Sandra takes a deep breath, and then sighs. Not sure how to respond, I gaze out into the night, watching the trees swaying gently, and the shadows dancing across the snow. Time seems to slow. I am curious, but also concerned not to force the conversation. I sense she wants to share her story but is searching for the words, or the inner strength. I wait while Sandra concentrates on flattening the top of a jump. Then, with an audible inhalation, she breaks the silence and proceeds to tell me her story. Even as tears well in her eyes, Sandra continues to drive meaningfully, shaping pyramids in the snow.

A little over two years ago, her boyfriend had been a well-known and respected groomer driver and terrain park designer at this resort. Sandra smiles as she describes spending many evenings with him as he shaped and crafted the jumps, and taught her how to drive. But one afternoon he made an error of judgement and a young up-and-coming local skier was accidentally killed. Although not directly his fault, many questions were asked, and Sandra's boyfriend lost his job. Sandra's voice becomes shaky as she describes the emotional turmoil

interviewer and interviewee is non-hierarchical and when the interviewer is prepared to invest his or her own personal identity in the relationship' (p. 252). Sandra seemed to appreciate my willingness to share my past snowboarding experiences, and also appeared to 'feel affirmed and empowered from being genuinely listened to' (Sherman Heyl, 2002, p. 375).

However, I was also careful to clarify that, while I am a snowboarder, during the interview I must privilege my roles and responsibilities as a researcher. Clarity of roles is an important ethical issue: 'The role of the interviewer can involve a tension between a professional distance and a personal friendship' (Kvale, 2007, p. 29).

Towards sensual, affective and respectful interviewing: Recognising the interview as a multi-sensorial experience, I pay close attention to the non-verbal dimensions of the interview (e.g. body preceding the incident. When her partner's job was advertised, Sandra never considered applying. How could she possibly work in the same terrain park where all of this pain, guilt and death had happened? Despite her doubts, her boyfriend and friends at the resort strongly encouraged her to apply. She admits that the first few months were incredibly difficult, but she persevered and now gets immense pride and satisfaction from her job. A male voice booms through the radio, startling us both; Sandra is instructed to make her way to another part of the mountain. Before heading over, she drops me at the base of the mountain. We say our quick farewells, and stepping out into the darkness, I turn to look back up at the young woman sitting high in the cabin of this huge machine. I am filled with admiration and respect.

language, eye contact, smell) (Fontana & Frey, 1994). I also try to take note of changes in pitch, tone and volume, and listen to the silences in a conversation.

Drawing upon all of my senses, I recognised this as a highly affective and affecting moment for Sandra. Thus, rather than exerting my authority and trying to control the interview, I tried to create space for her agency within the exchange. Throughout the interview, I encouraged her to set the pace and direction of the discussion, and 'choose how "deep" to go in answering questions' (Sherman Heyl, 2002, p. 375).

FINAL THOUGHTS: INTERVIEWING BODIES IN PHYSICAL CULTURAL FIELDS

Research is a process that occurs through the medium of a person – 'the researcher is always inevitably present in the research' (Stanley & Wise, 1993, cited in Wheaton, 2002, p. 246). This is certainly true in critical studies of SPC. Many (though not all) SPC scholars approach their subject with an embodied understanding of cultural norms and values developed via past or present active participation. The strengths and limitations of studying sporting cultures from an insider's perspective have been the subject of much debate within the field (Donnelly, 2006; Evers, 2006; Wheaton, 2002). The challenges of negotiating multiple roles (e.g. critical researcher, active participant, feminist) in the field of ethnographic inquiry are also garnering increasing critical reflection (see Carrington, 2008; Olive & Thorpe, 2011; Wheaton, 2002). Upon embarking on my project on snowboarding culture, I could have been considered a cultural insider. Prior to commencing this study, I had already held many roles in the snowboarding culture (i.e. novice, highly committed or 'core' snowboarder) and industry (i.e. semi-professional athlete, snowboard instructor, terrain-park employee and journalist). While my physical abilities and knowledge about snowboarding initially gave me access to the culture and a head start in discerning relevant sources and developing rapport with new and pre-existing contacts in the field, my position in the culture changed over time and varied depending on location. For example, in some snowboarding communities, a few key pre-existing contacts with long-time local snowboarders helped access places, events and potential interviewees, whereas in other locations I was an outsider without any cultural connections. Moreover, the length of my project and the dynamic nature of the snowboarding culture also meant that, as my research progressed, I became further removed in terms of age and generation (i.e. clothing styles, language) from the majority of core participants (mostly in their late teens and early twenties). This was not necessarily detrimental to my research, but rather required different strategies for gaining access to key informants and building rapport with interviewees. Thus, the key issue here is not whether one approaches their study as a past or present (non)active participant, or conducts semi-structured or unstructured, individual or group, or face-to-face or electronic interviews, but rather the reflexivity of the researcher in terms of how their dynamic position in the sport or physical culture *and* the academy, and their movement between these fields, influences the many 'how-to' decisions throughout the interview investigation, ranging from the sample size to the theoretical analysis and representation of interview data.

Acknowledging that the researcher is also embodied, and reflexively exploring some of the bodily tensions that can occur within the interview, can also open up new areas of inquiry. The following dialogue, which occurred in a bar following a presentation to a group of top-level New Zealand snowboarding coaches and instructors about gender, race and (dis)ability issues in snowboarding culture, illuminates how some partici-pants make judgements about one's cultural authenticity and credibility based on their readings of the researching body:

> *Attendee*: You really raised some interesting questions in your presentation, and as you can tell from the debate afterwards, people have lots of different opinions on this stuff. But I think it really helped that you have street-cred.

Holly: Thanks ... Do you mind if I ask what you mean by street-cred?

Attendee: You know, you are a cute chick, and one of us, you are a snowboarder. We can tell just by looking at your shoes and the shirt you are wearing. If you had come in here wearing a business suit, we probably would have been like, 'who is this idiot' and walked out. (field notes, 2007)

This example illustrates the capricious nature of some of my interactions with participants. While I made attempts to manage my impressions as a researcher (e.g. always being professional in my interactions with participants) and a snowboarder (e.g. by wearing snowboard-specific clothing, employing snowboarding argot, sharing snowboarding experiences), I could not control the interpretations that others drew from my performances. In this sense, as Shilling (2003) notes, I was 'caught in a web of communication irrespective of individual intentions' (p. 85). The key point is that throughout my fieldwork and during my interviews, I consciously reflected on my shifting interpretive positions as an (increasingly less) active snowboarder and a white, heterosexual, middle class female researcher and academic from New Zealand, and how these roles influenced my relationships in the field through interactions with interviewees. While the focus of my work was the corporeal experiences of 'other' snowboarders, it is important to acknowledge that my own embodied snowboarding experiences – as a participant and researcher – influenced every phase of this study, from conducting participant observations and interviews to theorising, to representing my research (also see Giardina & Newman, 2011; Newman, 2011; Olive & Thorpe, 2011; Thorpe, Barbour, & Bruce, 2011).

In light of the recent sensual turn in the social sciences and humanities, scholars have begun to question the bias towards the visual in ethnography (e.g. Howes, 2003; Pink, 2010; Rodaway, 1994; Sparkes, 2009; Stoller, 1997). For Pink (2010), the process of sensory ethnography can help us account for 'multisensoriality' in both the 'lives of people who participate in our research' and 'our craft' (p. 1). While the visual has traditionally been privileged in ethnographic fieldwork, the bias in interviewing has been towards the verbal; interview 'data' typically consists of disembodied and decontextualised 'quotes' from transcripts. During interviews, however, I adopted a 'sensory ethnographic' sensitivity by paying particular attention to the bodies of participants (e.g. clothing, bodily deportment, smells), as well my own snowboarding and researching body. I also took note of the unique sights, as well as the sounds, smells, tastes and touch, within the various physical cultural spaces in which interviews were conducted. To facilitate more vivid recall of the multi-sensual aspects of the interview experience upon returning 'home' from the field, I also recorded detailed notes of some of the non-verbal, embodied, social and sensual dimensions of the interview experience, including uncomfortable silences, changes in body language, facial expressions (e.g. smiles, frowns) and, on the odd occasion, tears. Indeed, listening to my audio-recordings alongside my field notes evoked more multidimensional memories of my interviews typically conducted within socially, physically and sensually loaded phases of fieldwork.

Each of the locations I visited for this project posed different opportunities *and* challenges (e.g. language, localism, cultural access, accommodation, pre-existing contacts in the field, funding). According to Stoller (1997), the key to doing research in complex transnational spaces is 'suppleness of imagination' (p. 91). Thus, I responded and adapted flexibly to the unique conditions of each field, and remained open to a wide variety of relationships and interactions as they arose in various locations (e.g. on chairlifts, in snowboard shops, on buses). Different ethnographic methods and interview styles became more important when conducting research in some physical cultural spaces, and with some individuals, than others. Moreover, my interactions and rapport with interviewees varied considerably based on an array of variables, including the sex, age, nationality and personality of the interviewee, as well as the location in which the interview was conducted (e.g. a noisy café, a quiet office, a snow groomer). In this way, it was typically the 'circumstance that defined the method rather than the method defining the circumstance' (Amit, 2000, p. 11).

In 1970, Norman Denzin proclaimed that 'interviewing is not easy' (p. 186). More than four decades later, conducting ethical, reflexive and interactional interviews, interpreting and analysing interview 'data', and representing this knowledge in meaningful ways, remains a difficult task indeed, and one that should not be underestimated. While much can be learned from reading textbooks about research methods or hearing about the experiences of other scholars using similar techniques, the quality of an interview study rests largely on the 'craftsmanship of the researcher':

> The openness of the interview, with its many on-the-spot decisions, puts strong demands on advance preparation and interviewer competence. The absence of a prescribed set of rules for interviewing creates an open-ended field of opportunity for the interviewer's skills, knowledge and intuition. (Kvale, 2007, p. 34)

Of course, there is a range of ways in which interviews can help produce socially meaningful and insightful analyses of particular dimensions of contemporary SPCs. My use of interviews has been inspired by the innovative and sensitive work of many critical sociologists of sport (e.g. Silk,

2002; Wheaton, 2002). In my field of ethnographic enquiry, however, I drew upon my own intuition and social skills, and developed my own set of rules for interviewing snowboarders. Thus, while I hope that the insights gleaned from my postmodern-inspired approach to interviewing prove useful for others embarking on their own projects, this chapter is by no means a prescriptive account of how to use qualitative interviews. Indeed, I look forward to seeing other sports scholars embrace the 'open-ended field of opportunity', and adopting more creative, reflexive, ethical and embodied approaches to interviewing in SPCs in global and/or local contexts.

FIVE KEY READINGS

1. Amis, J. (2005). Interviewing for case study research. In D. Andrews, D. Mason & M. Silk (Eds.), *Qualitative methods in sports studies* (pp. 104–138). Oxford: Berg.
This chapter provides a good overview of the various types of individual and group interviews that have been used within sports studies, and discusses some of the ethical, practical and political issues related to each of these approaches. This chapter also offers a number of exemplar studies from the field of sport and physical cultural studies that provide pointers towards good interviewing practice.

2. Fontana, A., & Frey, J. (2004). The interview: From structured questions to negotiated text. In N. Denzin & Y. Lincoln (Eds.), *Handbook of qualitative research* (2nd ed., pp. 645–670). London: Sage.
This chapter provides a thorough overview of the major types of quantitative and qualitative interviewing (structured, group, semi-structured and unstructured) used in the social sciences and humanities. The authors also discuss considerations for gendered interviewing, as well as issues of interpretation and reporting, and ethics.

3. Kvale, S., & Brinkmann, S. (2009). *InterViews: Learning the craft of qualitative research interviewing* (2nd ed.). London: Sage.
This text provides novice and experienced researchers with an accessible and engaging overview of the many practical, epistemological and ethical issues involved in interviewing. To further bring these issues to life, the text provides numerous examples, practical and conceptual assignments, and 'tool boxes'.

4. Oakley, A. (1981). Interviewing women: A contradiction in terms. In H. Roberts (Ed.), *Doing Feminist Research.* **London: Routledge.**
In this trailblazing article, Oakley identifies the many gaps between textbook 'recipes' for interviewing and her experiences as an interviewer studying women's experiences of motherhood during the late 1970s. Oakley's feminist critique of the traditional, masculinist, hierarchical approach to interviewing was integral to the 'revolutionising' of qualitative interviewing. Many of her arguments continue to have relevance today. Thus, all scholars seeking to conduct ethical, reflexive, respectful, interactional interviews in sport and physical cultural contexts would do well to go back to this highly original and interesting source.

5. Roulston, K. (2010). Considering quality in qualitative interviewing. *Qualitative Research, 10*(2), 199–228.
This article offers a valuable typology for understanding how theory informs the practice of qualitative interviewing from developing research questions to representing 'data'. Roulston (2010) identifies six theoretical approaches to interviewing– neo-positivist, romantic, constructionist, post-modern, transformative and decolonising – and explains how quality might be demonstrated from each perspective. This article will encourage emerging researchers to think critically about how theory implicitly and explicitly influences their approach to interviewing.

REFERENCES

Alversson, M. (2002). *Postmodernism and social research.* Buckingham: Open University Press.
Amis, J. (2005). Interviewing for case study research. In D. Andrews, D. Mason & M. Silk (Eds.), *Qualitative methods in sports studies* (pp. 104–138). Oxford: Berg.
Amit, V. (Ed.). (2000). *Constructing the field: Ethnographic fieldwork in the contemporary world.* Florence, Italy: Routledge.
Andrews, D., Mason, D., & Silk, M. (Eds.). (2005). *Qualitative methods in sports studies.* Oxford: Berg.
Atkinson, P., & Coffey, A. (2003). Revisiting the relationship between participant observation and interviewing. In J. Holstein & J. Gubrium (Eds.), *Inside interviewing: New lenses, new concerns* (pp. 415–428). Sage: London.
Baert, P. (2004). Pragmatism as philosophy of the social sciences. *European Journal of Social Theory, 7*(3), 355–369.
Bourdieu, P., & Wacquant, L. J. D. (1992). The purpose of reflexive sociology. In P. Bourdieu & L. J. D. Wacquant (Eds.), *An invitation to reflexive sociology* (pp. 61–215). Cambridge: Polity Press.

Burawoy, M., Blum, J. A., George, S., Gille, Z., Gowan, T., Haney, L., ... Thayer, M. (Eds.). (2000). *Global ethnography: Forces, connection, and imaginations in a postmodern world.* Berkeley, LA: University of California Press.

Carrington, B. (2008). 'What's the footballer doing here?' Racialized performativity, reflexivity and identity. *Cultural Studies ⇔ Critical Methodologies, 8*(4), 493–506.

de Castella, T. (2011, September 2). Why state surveys asked about bras and haddock. *BBC News Magazine.* Retrieved from http://www.bbc.co.uk/news/magazine-14746750. Accessed on December 12, 2011.

Denzin, N. (1970). *The research act.* Chicago, IL: Aldine.

Denzin, N. (1978). *The research act: A theoretical introduction to sociological methods.* New York: McGraw-Hill.

Denzin, N. (2001). The reflexive interview and a performative social science. *Qualitative Research, 1*(1), 23–46.

Denzin, N., & Lincoln, Y. (Eds.). (2011). *The SAGE handbook of qualitative research.* London: Sage.

Donnelly, M. (2006). Studying extreme sport: Beyond the core participants. *Journal of Sport and Social Issues, 30*, 219–224.

Ellis, C., & Berger, L. (2002). Their story/my story/our story: Including the researcher's experience in interview research. In J. Gubrium & J. Holstein (Eds.), *Handbook of interview research: Context and method* (pp. 849–876). London: Sage.

Evers, C. (2006). How to surf. *Journal of Sport and Social Issues, 30*(3), 229–243.

Fontana, A. (2002). Postmodern trends in interviewing. In J. Gubrium & J. Holstein (Eds.), *Handbook of interview research: Context and method* (pp. 161–175). London: Sage.

Fontana, A., & Frey, J. (1994). Interviewing: The art of science. In N. Denzin & Y. Lincoln (Eds.), *Handbook of qualitative research* (pp. 361–376). London: Sage.

Fontana, A., & Frey, J. (2000). The interview: From structured questions to negotiated text. In N. Denzin & Y. Lincoln (Eds.), *Handbook of qualitative research,* (pp. 645–670). London: Sage.

Fontana, A., & Prokos, A. (2007). *The interview: From formal to postmodern.* Walnut Creek, CA: Left Coast Press.

Giardina, M., & Newman, J. (2011). Physical cultural studies and embodied research acts. *Cultural Studies ⇔ Critical Methodologies, 11*(6), 523–534.

Holstein, J. A., & Gubrium, J. F. (2003). Inside interviewing: New lenses, new concerns. In J. Holstein & J. Gubrium (Eds.), *Inside interviewing: New lenses, new concerns* (pp. 3–30). London: Sage.

Howes, D. (2003). *Sensual relations: Engaging the senses in culture and social theory.* Michigan: University Press.

Kvale, S. (2007). *Doing interviews.* London: Sage.

Markula, P., & Pringle, R. (2006). *Foucault, sport and exercise: Power, knowledge and transforming the self.* London: Routledge.

Markula, P., & Silk, M. (2011). *Qualitative research for physical culture.* Basingstoke, Hampshire: Palgrave Macmillan.

Mason, J. (2002). *Qualitative researching* (2nd ed.). London: Sage.

Mills, C. W. (1959). *The sociological imagination.* Oxford: Oxford University Press.

Munslow, A. (2006). *Deconstructing history* (2nd ed.). London: Routledge.

Newman, J. (2011). [Un]comfortable in my own skin: Articulation, reflexivity, and the duality of self. *Cultural Studies ⇔ Critical Methodologies, 11*(6), 545–557.

Oakley, A. (1981). Interviewing women: A contradiction in terms. In H. Roberts (Ed.), *Doing feminist research*. Boston, MA: Routledge.

Oakley, A. (2003). Interviewing women: A contradiction in terms. In Y. Lincoln & N. Denzin (Eds.), *Turning points in qualitative research: Tying knots in a handkerchief* (pp. 243–264). Walnut Creek, CA: Altamira Press.

Olesen, V. (2011). Feminist qualitative research in the Millenium's first decade: Developments, challenges and prospects. In N. Denzin & Y. Lincoln (Eds.), *The SAGE handbook of qualitative research* (pp. 129–146). London: Sage.

Olive, R., & Thorpe, H. (2011). Negotiating the f-word in the field: Doing feminist ethnography in action sport cultures. *Sociology of Sport Journal, 28*, 421–440.

Pink, S. (2010). *Doing sensory ethnography*. Los Angeles: Sage.

Platt, J. (2002). The history of the interview. In J. Gubrium & J. Holstein (Eds.), *Handbook of interview research: Context and method* (pp. 33–54). London: Sage.

Rapley, T. (2001). The art(fullness) of open-ended interviewing: Some considerations on analysing interviews. *Qualitative Research, 1*(3), 303–323.

Rapley, T. (2004). Interviews. In C. Seale, G. Gobo, J. Gubrium & D. Silverman (Eds.), *Qualitative research practice* (pp. 15–33). London: Sage.

Richardson, L. (1992). Trash on the corner: Ethics and technology. *Journal of Contemporary Ethnography, 21*, 103–119.

Rodaway, P. (1994). *Sensuous geographies: Body, space and place*. London: Routledge.

Roulston, K. (2010). Considering quality in qualitative interviewing. *Qualitative Research, 10*(2), 199–228.

Seale, C. (1998). Qualitative interviewing. In C. Seale (Ed.), *Researching society and culture*. London: Sage.

Sherman Heyl, B. (2002). Ethnographic interviewing. In P. Atkinson, A. Coffey, S. Delamont, J. Lofland & L. Lofland (Eds.), *Handbook of ethnography* (pp. 369–383). London: Sage.

Shilling, C. (2003). *The body and social theory* (2nd ed.). London: Sage.

Silk, M. (2002). Bangsa Malaysia: Global sport, the city and the refurbishment of local identities. *Media, Culture and Society, 24*, 771–790.

Silverman, D. (1997). *Qualitative research: Theory, method and practice*. London: Sage.

Sin, C. H. (2003). Interviewing in 'place': The socio-spatial construction of interview data. *Area, 35*(3), 305–312.

Sparkes, A. (2009). Ethnography and the senses: Challenges and possibilities. *Qualitative Research in Sport and Exercise, 1*(1), 21–35.

Stoller, P. (1997). *Sensuous scholarship*. Philadelphia, PA: University of Pennsylvania Press.

Thorpe, H. (2011). *Snowboarding bodies in theory and practice*. Basingstoke, Hampshire: Palgrave Macmillan.

Thorpe, H., Barbour, K., & Bruce, T. (2011). Feminist journeys: Playing with theory and representation in physical cultural fields. *Sociology of Sport Journal, 28*, 106–134.

Wheaton, B. (2002). Babes on the beach, women in the surf: Researching gender, power and difference in the windsurfing culture. In J. Sugden & A. Tomlinson (Eds.), *Power games: A critical sociology of sport* (pp. 240–266). London: Routledge.

Wright, K. H. (2001). 'What's going on?' Larry Grossberg on the status quo of cultural studies: An interview. *Cultural Values, 5*(2), 133–162.

CHAPTER 4

NARRATIVE ANALYSIS IN SPORT AND PHYSICAL CULTURE

Brett Smith and Andrew C. Sparkes

ABSTRACT

Purpose – *The purpose of this chapter is to outline what narrative inquiry entails, why it is relevant for the study of sport and physical culture and how researchers might engage in its analytical methods.*

Design/methodology/approach – *Narrative inquiry as an approach, not simply a method, is delineated in this chapter. The design of a project is outlined. Three types of narrative analysis – holistic-content, holistic-form and meta-autoethnography – are the focus. The chapter also attends to the benefits of using multiple forms of analysis and representation as part of engaging with the methodology of crystallisation.*

Findings – *Key findings of narrative research on sport and physical culture are illuminated throughout.*

Research limitations/implications – *The limitations of narrative analysis are highlighted, including how in many narrative studies the interactional dynamics of storytelling are often neglected.*

Originality/value – *The chapter provides a succinct introduction to why narratives matter, how narrative analysis as a craft might be practised and what theoretical assumptions underpin it. The authors also highlight innovative practices for deepening understandings of sport and physical*

Qualitative Research on Sport and Physical Culture
Research in the Sociology of Sport, Volume 6, 79–99
ISSN: 1476-2854/doi:10.1108/S1476-2854(2012)0000006007

*culture. These include time-lining, mobile interviewing, analytical brack-
eting, crystallisation, meta-autoethnography and analysis as movement of
thought.*

Keywords: Story; narrative analysis; interviewing; visual methods;
crystallisation; meta-autoethnography

In recent years, as part of the 'narrative turn' in the social sciences (Crossley,
2000; Gubrium & Holstein, 2008), scholars have begun to treat seriously the
view that people structure experience through stories, and that a person is
essentially a storytelling animal. This has led to a sophisticated appreciation
of people as active social beings and focused attention on the way personal
and cultural realities are constructed through narrative and storytelling.
Such a narrative perspective is of some relevance to researchers in sport and
physical culture (SPC) who, as a group of professionals, are in the business
of dealing with a certain kind of 'experience'. As Sparkes and Partington
(2003) remind us, in both practice and for investigative purposes, we often
ask athletes to share with us their personal accounts of key moments or
phases in their career. In so doing, we are inviting stories. Thus, for example,
we have stories of winning against the odds, stories of heroic losses, injury
stories and 'comeback' stories, stories of anxiety and 'choking', and stories
of moments when everything comes together and we experience the
sensation of flow. Indeed, both athletes and researchers swim in a sea of
sporting stories and tales that we hear or read or listen to or see. As such,
there is much to be gained from engaging in the debate that surrounds the
narrative turn in other disciplines.

This chapter first introduces what narrative analysis is and highlights why
it is relevant for SPC. Next, how a narrative project might be designed is
considered. Following this, we describe how several kinds of narrative
analyses may be accomplished. The chapter ends by outlining several
strengths and weaknesses of narrative analysis as well as suggesting some
possible directions researchers might consider in the future.

WHAT IS NARRATIVE ANALYSIS AND WHY IS IT RELEVANT FOR SPC?

Narrative analysis is an umbrella term for an eclectic mix of methods for
making sense of, interpreting and representing data that have in common a

storied form (Smith & Sparkes, 2009a, 2009b; Sparkes, 2005). It takes stories and/or storytelling as its primary source of data and examines the content, structure, performance or context of the story or storytelling as a whole. The analytical interest is not simply in what is said in a story in terms of content. The language and telling itself is also examined along with the environments that give shape to narrative content, structure and performance. That is, in a narrative analysis the interest moves between *what* is being said and *how* and *why* a person or group tells and performs the story as they do in certain places under specific conditions. For example, the narrative analyst is interested in how a story is put together to convey meaning, namely, to make particular points to an audience. For whom was this story constructed, and for what purpose? What particular capacities of a story does the storyteller seek to utilise? Why is the sequence of events structured that way, and not another? What narrative resources from the cultural menu does the storyteller draw on, take for granted or ignore? Where do these resources derive from, and under what circumstances and conditions? Are there gaps and inconsistencies in storytelling that might suggest preferred, alternative or counter-narratives? What does the story say and do on, for and with people? How do listeners or readers respond to a story, with what affects and on whom (Riessman, 2008)?

In recent years, narrative analysis has garnered much interest among researchers studying SPC. Examining the history of why this has been the case, Smith (2010) highlighted that, for some researchers, narrative analyses offered a philosophically credible alternative way of doing research when faced with feeling disenchanted with post-positivism and methods that purport to produce theory-free knowledge. However, he also noted that, for others, there was more a pull than push towards narrative analyses for the benefits they can offer our understandings of SPC. This includes the ability to reveal the complexity of people's subjective worlds and the temporal, emotional and contextual quality of their lives. Others, such as Sparkes and Partington (2003), have been drawn to this approach because it allows them to address the experiential dynamics of involvement in sport and physical activity in a way that asks different questions and provides different insights than those provided by more traditional approaches.

Within our research on men who have suffered a catastrophic spinal cord injury (SCI) through playing sport and are now disabled, we have demonstrated that *narrative* is central to the process of attributing meaning to bodily experience over time and understanding physical culture (e.g. Smith, in press; Smith & Sparkes, 2002, 2004, 2005, 2008, 2011; Sparkes & Smith, 2002, 2003, 2008, 2011, 2012). It is central because meaning is

gaining knowledge through storytelling (winning, losing, heroics, injury, etc.)

constituted through narratives, and these very narratives are both embodied in and derived from culture. For example, drawing on Frank (1995), we highlight that in making sense of experiences of a sporting SCI, the participants not only tell stories *about* their bodies, they also tell stories *out of* and *through* their bodies.

In our work on SCI and SPC, we have also stressed that the body is not free to construct just *any* story it wishes about itself. In the first instance, it is constrained by its fleshy physicality. Furthermore, while people construct stories in personally meaningful ways and act to defend a sense of personal authenticity, the stories a body tells are given meaning and constructed from the cultural menu of narrative resources that are made available to them. For example, environments like the family, physical education classes, sporting organisations or rehabilitation institutions provide narrative resources people use to make up and tell stories. As such, no story is entirely ever anyone's own or constructed solely by them. It is co-constructed by people in relational networks and creatively borrows from the narratives that pre-exist them and already circulate in society and culture. What is more, these narratives, as actors outside us (Frank, 2010), have the capacity to *do* things on and for us. This includes performing the work of teaching bodies who they ought to be, who they might like to be and who they can be. It also involves connecting and disconnecting bodies, institutions, products, images, emotions and other stories. Conceptualised in these ways, narrative analyses hold onto understanding the sporting body as not just material or subjective, but also culturally produced and producing, with narratives from culture doing 'positive' and 'dangerous' work on and for bodies.

Furthermore, in some recent work, we have highlighted the centrality of narrative, and its relevance to SPC, through the concepts of 'narrative interpellation' (Griffin, 2010) and 'narrative habitus' (Frank, 2010). Here, we suggested that sporting bodies are also interpellated – 'hailed'/called – by certain narratives to acknowledge and respond to cultural ideologies to be certain individuals as subjects when they experience life-threatening illness (Sparkes, Perez-Samaniego, & Smith 2012), become impaired (Smith, in press) or choose to become mature bodybuilders (Phoenix & Smith, 2011). The narrative habitus, it was argued in these three cases, is an unchosen force in any choice to be interpellated by certain narratives and not others. Narrative habitus is an acquired embodied disposition formed in the context of people's social locations to hear some stories as those that one should listen to, should tell, should be guided by or should pass over. It describes the embedding of stories in bodies and the embodied sense of attraction, indifference or repulsion that people feel in response to stories that leads them to define a certain story as for them or not.

For example, in our work with an elite male athlete (David) who was diagnosed with cancer that eventually led to his death, we highlight the ways in which due to the narrative habitus he developed via his socialisation into sport, David was drawn towards the dominant cultural story in Western cultures relating to illness and recovery (the restitution narrative). Our analysis also revealed that he has a strong affinity for the narrative map provided by the published autobiography of Lance Armstrong who 'defeated' cancer and made a successful comeback to elite sport. We suggest that, in combination, these operate as actors to frame David's experiences of illness, and influenced the process by which he made social comparisons with other cancer patients and athletes in ways that locked him into certain stories that he felt were 'right' for him while ignoring other possible storylines that were not deemed relevant in terms of his narrative habitus. As such, our analysis provides an exemplar of how the corporeal body and the meanings given to it are powerfully shaped by the narrative resources provided by the wider culture and also how certain kinds of bodies have elective affinities for certain kinds of narratives over others.

DOING NARRATIVE ANALYSIS

There are many ways to plan and execute a narrative analysis. Here is a flavour that we hope will help with going about designing an SPC project.

Animating Interest

A researcher interested in SPC will need to craft a research purpose and a series of research questions around it. But before doing this, be as clear as possible about the fundamental interest (Frank, 2012). What has animated our work on catastrophic SCI and SPC for the first five years was this: What happens to people who have invested a great deal in developing a sporting body and then, due to sustaining an SCI playing sport, move from a culturally valued able body to a disabled body less valued in our culture? Out of this animating interest, our recent starting point for research has moved to the following issue: Disabled persons' health and well-being is too often damaged; why is this, and how could it change? Being as clear as possible about our fundamental interest has been invaluable. It is what we return to when we are confused. It helps us get things moving again when our research on SPC loses its way.

Collecting Stories

Autobiographies, letters, vignettes, newspapers, ethnographic fieldwork notes and visual material (like photographs and DVDs) can all be sources of stories. We have used all of these in our SPC research on SCI and found them to be excellent sources for collecting stories. But the primary source we have used is the life story interview (Atkinson, 2007). The life story interview, or what is sometimes called a narrative interview (Crossley, 2000), is concerned with inviting participants to tell stories about their life. The life interview moves from a semi-structured format towards an unstructured format as the interview unfolds over time. This is because it puts greater emphasis on inviting life stories in the participants' own words and recounting events in their preferred order without asking them too many direct and predetermined questions. What differentiates a life story interview from many types of interview is that stories are purposefully invited rather than letting them happen. The interest is on stories as opposed to collecting relatively thin descriptions, evaluations, reports, technical accounts or other kinds of discourse from participants.

To collect stories in an interview, it can be useful to simply ask for stories: for example, 'Can you tell me a story about your childhood'? However, inviting life stories and sustaining a narrative can be difficult. It not only requires participants who can and wish to tell stories, but also a skilled and active interviewer. Here are some 'tips' we have gleaned over the years from our SPC work for inviting and sustaining stories (see also Sparkes & Smith, forthcoming). They are not exhaustive and interviewers should adapt them according to the specific experiences of the interviewees:

- Orientate yourself to the participant as someone who *is* a storyteller as opposed to a vessel to extract information out of. To help with *orientation*, appreciate that participants' stories are for another just as much as for them, and that what is spoken is a relationship in which you are not separate from but implicated in.
- Ask your participant to imagine their life as an unfinished book (see Crossley, 2000). Ask them to divide their life into its major chapters, and briefly describe each chapter. Ask them to give a name to each chapter and describe the content of each. You might enquire into who the

characters are in each chapter, what the central theme(s) or message(s) of the book is (are) about and what might future chapters contain. Discuss what makes for a transition from one chapter to the next. Also you could discuss whom they would share the book with, hide it from, and say needs to read it. You could examine how they could have told a different story about their life and what that other story could be. Whatever the case, remember that in order to invite stories, you need to talk less and listen more. It is your participant's tales you want to hear and learn from.

- To help people answer you more readily and more fully, sometimes ask questions in somewhat broken syntax, with a hesitant tone indicating that you are unsure of your vocabulary. Trail off your interview voice at the end of questions, often not completing the grammatical form of the question. What your broken questions can convey is openness for them to tell you their stories.
- Sometimes, in specific contexts and for certain purposes, adopt the strategy that Dowling & Flintof (2011) termed 'antagonistic interviewing'. In this type of interview, researchers seek to challenge certain stories so that space is created for alternative or more complex storylines to emerge.
- At times collect life stories also using 'mobile interviewing' (Brown & Durrheim, 2009). In this kind of interview, rather than two bodies sitting down in the participant's home as is often the case in interviewing, the researcher interviews the participant as they move together through spaces the participant chooses. Mobile interviewing is especially well suited to research on SPC as the physical and sensorial bodies move in and through the places that are significant to the participant as they direct where and how you move. This can provoke contextually meaningful stories that may not have been produced in a 'sedentary' interview. It also creates a space where participants have more control over the stories they tell. This can be particularly useful when dealing with sensitive topics or areas that might pose a threat to a participant's embodied senses of self or sporting identity.
- To become a better interviewer, examine the transcribed data for how you yourself – as the interviewer – invited and sustained stories (or not). To help with this, ask such questions as: What type of questions did I ask? Did I flood the interview with academic jargon or social scientific categories? How did I relate to the participant? How did the participant and I work together to enable or constrain storytelling? During turn-taking exchanges when talking, which stories were advanced or suppressed, and how?
- Consider visual or graphic elicitation techniques to invite richer or different stories (see Phoenix, 2010; Sparkes & Smith – see Chapter 8).

Visual techniques include photo elicitation. This involves using photographs to invoke memory and elicit stories from participants in the course of an interview. Among the different kinds of graphic elicitation methods, time-lining has also proved useful. This is a visual method in which a participant and/or researcher draws a temporal plot about a specific subject (e.g. weight loss), linking events along the way, in order to visually represent experience of the subject matter as it unfolded over time. The time-line drawn is then used to elicit further stories about the participants' life and cultural physicality.

Deciding What is a Story

Having sought to invite stories in an interview, or collected them via fieldwork or from the Internet, for example, what segments of speech, visual material, writing or bodily enactment count as stories for analysis? Narrative analysis raises the thorny question of just what is a story? Not all talk, images, text or bodily performances that are collected constitute a story.

Definitions proliferate about just what a 'story' is. One useful way suggested by Frank (2012) to think about stories is to imagine them horizontally, vertically and from the perspective of a child. On a horizontal dimension, unfolding in real time, stories have a minimum of a *complicating action* and a *resolution* to the complication. Complicating action is the core of the story that tells the audience 'Then what happened?' through the use of a temporal juncture. The resolution or result tells the audience 'what finally happened'. Vertically, stories have enough of the aspects that include characters, suspense or trouble, imagination, point of view, evaluation and a settings/context (Frank, 2012). What is *enough* can be determined by an experience-centred approach to narrative (Squire, 2008), or what Frank termed 'the bedtime test'. If a child wants to hear a story before bed, a story has to make the complication action suspenseful, and this, according to Frank, usually hinges on the strengths and flaws of the characters who deal with the complication. Further, he noted, when a story is told to someone (e.g. a child before bed), it should remain recognisable across multiple (re)tellings and relate to human experience.

Adopting a comparative approach, we have also found that appreciating what does *not* count as a story has been useful in helping us to better understand what constitutes a story for the purposes of SPC research. Wendgraf (2001), for example, compares narrative to the following four discourses: *descriptions* – the assertion that particular entities have properties, yet in a timeless non-historical way. No attempt is made at storytelling/narration; *arguments* – the development of argument and theorising and position taking, typically from a present-time perspective; *reports* – a form in which a sequence of events, experiences and action is recounted, but in a relatively experience-thin manner and *evaluations* – the 'moral of the story'. Moreover, Tilly (2006) differentiated between *technical accounts* and stories. Technical accounts might often take a narrative form in that the events follow in sequential order, with some causal relation between them, but technical accounts depend on specialised knowledge and language authorised by experts. Stories are, however, 'non-specialised' (Frank, 2012, p. 41).

NARRATIVE ANALYSES

In dedicating a section to analysis at this stage in the chapter, there is the danger of presenting analysis as if it begins after collecting data and deciding on what is a story, and then stops before writing up the research. But this is not how narrative analysis works, or should work. First, data collection and analysis proceed in an *iterative* fashion, each informing each other. That is to say, data collection and analysis occur concurrently during the research process. Second, an understanding of what is a story is not set in stone. It is possible you might revise your decisions on what it is as you hear more stories or read more literature. Third, for narrative researchers, writing is not something done at the end of the project. Rather than 'writing up' what has already been found, researchers write continuously and creatively throughout the research. There is good reason for this. Analysis takes place in the process of writing, and thus writing is a form of analysis (Frank, 2012; Richardson, 2000; Sparkes, 2002). Because of this conjunction of analysis and writing, it is recommended that researchers start writing early and revise, edit and revise their research report along the way. We have certainly found that in our own work on SPC and SCI, a research paper starts as a series of notes and over a series of months, sometimes years as in one case (Smith & Sparkes, 2008), draft after draft is written as we work with stories collected and write to make sense of them.

But while analysis takes place in the process of writing, writing has to start somewhere. To get analysis moving, there are multiple methods to choose from. One way to work through these choices is using the degree to which empirical and analytical emphasis is placed on the *whats* (e.g. the storied content or what is a story about) as opposed to *hows* (e.g. how narratives are organised or performed). Analyses that focus primarily on the *whats* of stories include a holistic-content narrative analysis (Lieblich, Tuval-Mashiach, & Zilber 1998) and a narrative identity analysis (McAdams, 2010). Analyses that focus on the *hows* of narrative can be found in Gubrium and Holstein's (2008) discourse analysis of informed emphasis on narrative practice, Frank's (2012) dialogical narrative analysis and the structural analyses as described by Riessman (2008). Phoenix and Howe (2010) also used a narrative analysis to examine how context is played out in an athlete's story of injury. Finally, there are some analyses that emphasise the reflexive interplay between the *whats* and *hows* of storytelling, showing throughout a text both what is in a story and how it is organised, shaped by narrative environments and performed in relation to other bodies. An example here is the work of Sparkes and Partington (2003) who combine an interest with the *whats* of the flow experience as described in interviews with a concern for *how* this storytelling process is shaped by the gendered environment of a white water canoeing club.

In our own SPC research on SCI, we have used a variety of narrative analyses to examine the *whats* and *hows* of stories. Of course, one cannot focus on both the *whats* and *hows* at the same time. Analytically, this is just too demanding, and ultimately unproductive. The technique of *analytical bracketing* proved useful here. This is the process of analytically moving back and forth between the *whats* and *hows* of narrativity (Gubrium & Holstein, 2008). As analysis proceeds, the researcher alternatively orientates to the different aspects of stories and storytelling. Accordingly, at first in our research, we focused our attention on the *whats* of stories, such as what metaphors are being used, what times tenses are used to frame the story and what kinds of hope are invoked in the telling (Smith & Sparkes, 2004, 2005; Sparkes & Smith, 2003). In so doing, we analytically bracketed out any attention or concerns for *how* the stories were being told and how they were structured. One analysis we used to examine the content of the story was a holistic-content narrative analysis (Lieblich, Tuval-Mashiach, & Zilber, 1998)

The Whats of Narrative: A Holistic Analysis of Content

In this analysis, the interest is on examining the core pattern in the life story. Other analyses, such as a content analysis, provide a way in which researchers may conceptualise all the independent themes that are present in a narrative; they do not, however, provide a way for researchers to link those themes in relation to an evolving story. A holistic-content analysis does just this, and this is one of its key strengths. But, just how do researchers do this kind of narrative analysis? Adapting how Lieblich et al. (1998, pp. 62–63) set it out in light of our experiences of using a holistic-content analysis, our application of it to stories of SPC can be described as follows:

1. *Immersion*: Read the material and listen to recorded data repeatedly until a pattern emerges.
2. *Writing initial thoughts*: Write an initial first impression of the entire life story. Initial impressions in this report might include a general impression as to the core life story pattern as well as contradictions, unusual parts of the story, unfinished descriptions and issues that disturb the teller and the listener.
3. *Select foci of the story*: Identify specific themes to follow within the whole story. Storytellers often devote more time to important themes; however, omissions and brief references may also be critical to interpretation of a life story pattern. Weave and re-weave ideas gleaned from all this into your report. Edit and edit more.
4. *Interpreting themes*: Mark the various themes in the story, read them separately and repeatedly. Go beyond what is in the data (manifest content) and interpret it by drawing on theory and asking questions such as 'What is going on here?', 'What does this theme mean?', 'What are the assumptions underpinning it?', 'What are the implications of this theme?', 'What conditions are likely to have given rise to it?' and 'What is the overall story the different themes reveal about the topic?' Continue the process of writing, and thus analysis, by integrating and editing the report, remembering that each theme and interpretation must lead to a next part.
5. *Tracking within a narrative*: Keep track of your results in several ways, including following each theme throughout the story and noting conclusions. Also examine where a theme appears for the first and last time, the cross-over between themes, the context for each one, the main theme(s), marginal themes, the characters, predicament (a situation, sometimes unpleasant, trying, or troublesome) within each, and episodes that contradict themes in terms of content, mood, imagery and evaluations.
6. *Continue writing*: Write and re-write an integrated and vivid tale of the results. Ask yourself as you write what is stake for people in the representation you're writing: how will they be represented and with what possible affects? What are the ethics of the representational form chosen?

Having attended primarily to *what* was in the stories we collected using a holistic-content analysis, our next analytical move in our work on SCI and SPC was to bracket the *whats* in order to analyse the *hows*. This included examining the discrete stylistic or linguistic characteristics of defined units of the narrative through the use of a categorical-form mode of analysis (see Smith & Sparkes, 2004). Another analysis we used for the purpose of understanding how people respond to a certain kind of story was a dialogical narrative analysis as described by Frank (2012) (see Smith & Sparkes, 2011). But prior to using either of these, we first wanted to know about what narrative resources the participants were drawing on and how they organised their own stories. We thus used a structural form of analysis.

The Hows of Narrative: Holistic Analysis of Form

There are many kinds of structural analysis (Riessman, 2008; Sparkes, 2005). One used in our work on SPC was what Lieblich et al. (1998) termed a holistic-form narrative analysis. Like in a categorical-form analysis, the focus here is on the analysis of the narrative as a whole. But in this analysis, the goal is to demonstrate how narrative material may be used to learn about variations in structure (Lieblich et al., 1998). The interest is on how stories are put together and what kind of narrative is drawn on to help, like scaffold, structure the story being told. Here are some 'tips' to help go about doing a holistic-form narrative analysis.

1. *Immersion*: Read the material repeatedly.
2. *Writing initial thoughts*: Write an initial first impression of how the story is put together, making notes on the events, the sequence of them, characters involved and any sense of suspense.
3. *Identify the development of the plot*: Identify the axis of each stage and how the plot develops. This can involve noting in the margins of the transcript, for example, the beginning, middle and end of the story, noting in between how events are connected and how the story is told in relation to the person's past, present and future. Again, write your thoughts on how the plot develops. Edit the report in light of your thoughts.
4. *Identify the dynamics of the plot*: To help with this, you might also ask yourself such questions as, 'What narrative resources shape how the story is being told'? 'What kinds of stories are imposing themselves on the

person?' Inferring from particular forms of speech, and noting your inferences in the margins of the transcript, can also help with the process of identifying the dynamics of the plot. These forms may include the following:

(a) Reflections on specific phases in the interviewee's life.
(b) Responses to a query about why the interviewee chose to end a stage at a given point (indicated in answers to questions posed by interviewer).
(c) Use of terms that express the structural component of the narrative (e.g. 'crossroads', 'turning point').

5. *Interpretive retelling*: Practise telling the type of story you're hearing, as *if* it were your own. Again, write and re-write to keep the analysis moving: edit, and edit again.

6. *Develop a structural graph*: You may wish to depict the story you are hearing on a graph. For example, a story may be one of progress towards a certain goal or a much more messy series of 'up' and 'downs'.

7. *Build a typology*: Cluster stories into ideal types and structure your writing around them, revising and editing along the way to help 'discover' further the types of narratives used. For example, in our SPC work on SCI, we clustered the stories the men tell into three types: restitution, chaos and quest. One advantage of doing this is that no individual storyteller is stripped of their uniqueness or agency, while at the same time they are understood as drawing on types of narratives, as resources, to frame their lives.

Having offered a description of how a structural analysis and a holistic-content analysis might be done, it should be recognised that these descriptions should not been treated in formulaic or codified way. They are neither a discrete set of steps nor a formula to rigidly follow. In practice, a holistic-content or holistic-form analysis does not work like this, or should do. Analysis needs to be rigorous, but it is craft. In our work on SPC, we have sometimes jumped back and forth between each phase described. We also have relied on theoretical memos written throughout the process as well a reflexive journal. Further, our work has benefited from us operating as 'critical friends'. This is the process of dialogue. It involves a researcher (e.g. Brett) giving voice to their interpretations in relation to another person (e.g. Andrew) who listens and offers critical feedback. A researcher who acts as critical friend seeks to encourage reflection upon, and exploration of, alternative analytical explanations and

holistic analyses =

interpretations as they emerge in relation to the data and writing. As Wolcott (1994) put it:

> The crucial element in soliciting feedback seems to be to engage in dialogue about interpretive possibilities. As with writing, engaging in a dialogue requires that you first give voice to your thought processes. In the process of giving voice to your thoughts you give access to them as well. There is some subtle reciprocity involved here; you are never totally free to ignore the suggestions of invited critics ... Every invited reviewer is ... a potential source of insight into the adequacy of your descriptive account, the incisiveness of your analysis, the depth of your interpretation. Every opinion offered is also a reminder that for every additional viewer there is an additional view. (p. 42)

Acting as critical friends, and engaging in dialogue with each other as friends who trust each other in the traditional sense too, has helped not only develop our interpretations of the stories we have collected on SPC. This dialogical process has also opened up (further) the ways we *feel* our way into and out of analysis via the fullness of our sensual corporality (see Sparkes & Smith, 2012). To help understand this process better, as well as continue our aspiration to build a more complex picture of participant's lives and develop an embodied narrative analysis that shows, rather than tells, the reflexive interplay between the *whats* and *hows* of storytelling, we thus turned to the creative analytical practice (CAP) known as autoethnography.

The Whats and Hows of Narrative: Meta-Autoethnography and Crystallisation

What Richardson (2000) termed CAP is in inclusive term for those representational practices that include ethnographic creative non-fiction, poetry and performance texts (Sparkes, 2002). Autoethnography (see Chapter 9) is also an example of CAP. As defined by Ellis and Bochner (2000), autoethnography as an 'autobiographical genre of writing and research that displays multiple layers of consciousness, connecting the personal to the cultural' (p. 739). Because another chapter in this book is dedicated to this kind of CAP, we will not rehearse how it can be done or what it entails. Instead, it is tempting to revisit the autoethnography that both builds on our previous SCI and SPC research (Sparkes & Smith, 2012) and produces here a *meta-autoethnography*. Ellis (2009) described meta-autoethnographies as 'occasions in which I revisit my original representation, consider responses, and write an autoethnographic account about autoethnography' (p. 13). Thus, this chapter could have provided opportunities to alter the frame in which we wrote the original story, ask questions we didn't ask then, consider others' responses to the original story and include vignettes of related experiences that have happened since we experienced and wrote the story and now affect the way we look back at the story of SPC and SCI.

In addition, writing a meta-autoethnography could have had the benefit of developing further our engagement with a methodology of *crystallisation*. Building on the work of Richardson (2000), Ellingson (2009) described crystallisation as a methodology in which multiple forms of analysis and multiple genres of representation are combined in one of two ways. *Integrated crystallisation* brings together different analyses and forms of representation to produce a single text. This might, for example, occur in one book or Ph.D. dissertation. In contrast, our own work on SPC and SCI has evolved into what Ellingson termed *dendritic crystallisation*. This is the ongoing and dispersed process of making meaning of the same topic (e.g. SPC and SCI) through multiple forms of analysis and forms of representation to produce a series of related texts. For example, by using multiple narrative analyses as well as representing spinal injured person's stories through multiple genres, we have sought in different publications to build a rich and openly partial account of SCI and SPC that problematises its own construction, highlights our own vulnerabilities and positionality, makes claims about socially constructed meanings and reveals the indeterminacy of knowledge claims even as it makes them. We also hoped this dendritic crystallisation process would enable us to not only better reach across academic disciplines but also engage stakeholder audiences such as practitioners, policy makers and disability community organisations.

Accordingly, we could close this section on how to do analysis with the example of meta-autoethnography, thereby extending our engagement with dendritic crystallisation. Indeed, we believe meta-autoethnography to be an important addition to our analytical repertoire for studying not just what participants have to say about sporting physical cultures but also how we *ourselves* as researchers do work on this topic and are wrapped up in SCP. Despite its importance, right now any meta-autoethnography we would write might be a 'nice story', but it would have little to say that is worthwhile. Admitting this can be difficult in an academic culture where publishing is a major part of what counts to secure and keep a job. But, for us, sometimes it can be more productive to hold back from trying to publish a particular piece (sometimes for years), and in the meantime think with stories, write, read, edit and work through ideas, throwing many out, and revising others. And, of course, when possible enjoy this analytical process – it is often difficult, but it can be fun too!

[handwritten margin note: integrated = many analysis into one text dendritic = one topic through multiple texts.]

CONCLUSION

Narrative analysis as a family of methods that focus on stories and storytelling has much to offer (Smith & Sparkes, 2009a, 2009b). Many narrative analyses seek to combine an emphasis on people as agents of their behaviour and a humanistic image of the person alongside unpacking the cultural discursive practices that people often take for granted, but which play a key role in shaping our physical culture. When done well, narrative analyses do not reduce stories to inert material, left devoid of spirit, as often happens in many other qualitative analyses of lived experience. Narrative analysts strive to keep stories intact, hear how multiple voices find expression within any single story and make their reports vivid. Another strength of narrative analyses when done well is that, unlike many other kinds of analysis, they call on the researcher to commit to unfinalisability (Frank, 2012). This means respecting in analysis that stories of SPC always, like human lives that are spun through them, have the capacity to change and that as long as they are alive, bodies telling stories have not yet spoken their last word. A commitment to unfinalisability also means respecting that any ending to a research paper is provisional, not the final word on SPC (Frank, 2012).

Like any form of analysis, however, narrative analyses cannot do everything. First, many narrative analyses analyse stories collected from interviews. As a result, analysts can say little about way stories are actually composed in everyday talk and told in particular interactional contexts. Another 'limit is that if narrative analysis means following the stories, stories travel further – plots are borrowed and tropes resonate – than any one narrative analyst can pursue direct observation' (Frank, 2012, p. 40). Furthermore, many narrative analyses (purposefully) lack a prescribed set of steps that should be rigidly followed. For *some* researchers – and unfortunately *some* journal editors, journal reviewers, and thesis examiners and ethics committees – this equals 'unrigorous or unscientific research'.

However, such a view is an overly simplistic and narrow one of what methods mean. As Frank (2010) reminded us, methods can be comprehended as a canonical sequence of prescribed analytical steps. However, they can also legitimately be understood as a heuristic guide and craft. Such an understanding encourages *movement of thought*. As Frank stated: 'Too many methods seem to prevent thought from *moving*. Analytic or interpretive thought that is moving is more likely to allow and recognise movements in the thought being interpreted' (p. 73). Accordingly, narrative analysis needs to be understood as more of a craft for encouraging thought to move than a codified method with one set of prescribed steps to follow for finding what the method suggests they should.

With regards to the future of narrative analysis, there are many exciting challenges ahead. One of these is to re-address the methodological balance of how we collect and invite stories for analysis. Currently most narrative analyses, like most qualitative research, rely on interview data. This, in itself, is not 'bad' or 'wrong'. But the way stories are actually composed in everyday talk and told in particular interactional contexts cannot be understood. While not abandoning interviews, future research needs to adjust the methodological balance by using naturalistic data. This is data not provoked by the researcher. It refers to research materials of what people actually say and do that would (ideally) have been generated irrespective of the researcher's activities. Likewise, there is much narrative research that collects 'big stories', but very little within sport that also collects 'small stories' – the stories told during interaction, generally within everyday settings, about very mundane things and everyday occurrences. One rare sport example of an analysis that examined both 'big' and 'small' stories can be found in Phoenix and Sparkes (2009) who used this approach to explore how positive aging was performed in relation to sport and health behaviours. Another possible future direction for researchers to take in relation to narrative and sport is to examine the *different work* narratives *do* on, for and in physical culture. Finally, but by no means last, analyses of SPC might begin to engage with a methodology of crystallisation and reap the benefits that such an engagement can bring in terms of producing a highly rich and complex understanding of SPC.

Whatever direction researchers take, when done well narrative analyses have much to offer researchers interested in SPC. We hope this chapter acts as spur to further dialogue on the many ways narrative can enhance our knowledge and change people's lives.

FIVE KEY READINGS

1. Smith, B., & Sparkes, A. (2008). Changing bodies, changing narratives and the consequences of tellability: A case study of becoming disabled through sport. *Sociology of Health and Illness, 30*(2), 217–236.
This paper highlights a narrative analysis in action relative to SPC. It identifies one type of story a person lives by (the chaos narrative) and the work this story can have on and in a person. Numerous theories and

[margin handwritten note: good for sports as you can gain knowledge & actual experience]

concepts are woven throughout the paper, demonstrating the importance of interpreting stories as opposed to just describing them.

2. Smith, B., & Sparkes, A. (2011). Multiple responses to a chaos narrative. *Health: An Interdisciplinary Journal for the Social Study of Health, Illness & Medicine, 15*(1), 38–53.
This paper builds on the one above. It offers a new typology relative to disability and SPC for understanding how people respond to certain story (i.e. chaos) and the consequences these responses can have on disabled people. It focuses attention on both the story and listeners of this story as opposed to just the storyteller.

3. Phoenix, C., & Smith, B. (2011). Telling a (good?) counterstory of aging: Natural bodybuilding meets the narrative of decline. *The Journals of Gerontology Series B: Psychological Sciences and Social Sciences, 66*(5), 628–639.
This paper highlights several narrative analyses in action and describes what theoretically underpins these analyses. In relation to SPC, the paper demonstrates how mature, natural bodybuilders spin stories of their lives in different ways to resist in varying degrees the negative views of aging. The potential of narrative for changing human lives and behaviour across the life course in more positive and nuanced ways is also highlighted.

4. Griffin, M. (2010). Setting the scene: Hailing women into a running identity. *Qualitative Research in Sport & Exercise, 2*, 153–174.
This paper demonstrates a narrative visual analysis, noting how it can be done and showing what it can achieve for understanding SPC. New concepts are developed. Readers are taken vividly into the worlds of women's physical culture via multiple visual materials, running stories and strong interpretations. The analysis shows that researchers must also examine narratives as visual and not simply as verbal discourses.

5. Sparkes, A., Perez-Samaniego, V., & Smith, B. (2012). Social comparison processes, narrative mapping, and their shaping of the cancer experience: A case study of an elite athlete. *Health: An Interdisciplinary Journal for the Social Study of Health, Illness & Medicine, 16*(5), 467–488.
This paper demonstrates how a narrative analysis can creatively combine a concern for both *what* is said in the story told and *how* it is said under certain circumstances. It also illustrates the *work* that stories *do* as actors in shaping the experiences of the individual teller and vividly illuminates the

intimate relationship that personal stories have with the cultural context in which they are constructed and performed in relation to specific kinds of narrative maps that are available for consumption. The holding power of certain stories to crowd out and silence other stories in ways that can be both enabling and constraining for individuals and groups is also made evident.

REFERENCES

Atkinson, R. (2007). The life story interview as a bridge in narrative inquiry. In D. J. Clandidnin (Ed.), *Handbook of narrative inquiry* (pp. 224–245). London: Sage.

Brown, L., & Durrheim, K. (2009). Different kinds of knowing: Generating qualitative data through mobile interviewing. *Qualitative Inquiry, 15*, 911–993.

Crossley, M. (2000). *Introducing narrative psychology*. Buckingham: Open University Press.

Dowling, F., & Flintof, A. (2011). Getting beyond normative interview talk of sameness and celebrating difference. *Qualitative Research in Sport, Exercise, & Health, 3*, 63–79.

Ellingson, L. (2009). *Engaging crystallisation in qualitative research*. London: Sage.

Ellis, C. (2009). *Revision: Autoethnographic reflections on life and work*. Walnut Creek, CA: Left Coast.

Ellis, C., & Bochner, A. P. (2000). Autoethnography, personal narrative, reflexivity. In N. Denzin & Y. Lincoln (Eds.), *Handbook of qualitative research* (2nd ed., pp. 733–768). London: Sage.

Frank, A. W. (1995). *The wounded storyteller*. Chicago, IL: The University of Chicago Press.

Frank, A. W. (2010). *Letting stories breathe*. Chicago, IL: The University of Chicago Press.

Frank, A. W. (2012). Practicing dialogical narrative analysis. In J. Holstein & J. Gubrium (Eds.), *Varieties of narrative analysis* (pp. 33–52). London: Sage.

Griffin, M. (2010). Setting the scene: Hailing women into a running identity. *Qualitative Research in Sport & Exercise, 2*, 153–174.

Gubrium, J., & Holstein, J. (2008). *Analysing narrative reality*. London: Sage.

McAdams, D. (2012). Exploring psychological themes through life-narrative accounts. In J. Holstein & J. Gubrium (Eds.), *Varieties of narrative analysis* (pp. 15–32). London: Sage.

Lieblich, A., Tuval-Mashiach, R., & Zilber, T. (1998). *Narrative research: Reading, analysis, and interpretation*. London: Sage.

Phoenix, C. (2010). Seeing the world of physical culture: The potential of visual methods for qualitative research in sport and exercise. *Qualitative Research in Sport & Exercise, 2*, 93–108.

Phoenix, C., & Howe, A. (2010). Working the when, where, and who of social context: The case of a traumatic injury narrative. *Qualitative Research in Psychology, 7*, 140–155.

Phoenix, C., & Smith, B. (2011). Telling a (good?) counterstory of aging: Natural bodybuilding meets the narrative of decline. *The Journals of Gerontology Series B: Psychological Sciences and Social Sciences, 66*, 628–639.

Phoenix, C., & Sparkes, A. (2009). Being Fred: Big stories, small stories and the accomplishment of a positive ageing identity. *Qualitative Research, 9*, 83–99.

Riessman, C. (2008). *Narrative methods for the human sciences*. London: Sage.

Richardson, L. (2000). Writing: A method of inquiry. In N. Denzin & Y. Lincoln (Eds.), *Handbook of qualitative research* (2nd ed., pp. 923–948). London: Sage.

Smith, B. (2010). Narrative inquiry: Ongoing conversations and questions for sport psychology research. *International Review of Sport Psychology, 3*, 87–107.

Smith, B. (in-press). Disability, sport, and men's narratives of health: A qualitative study. *Health Psychology.*

Smith, B., & Sparkes, A. (2004). Men, sport, and spinal cord injury: An analysis of metaphors and narrative types. *Disability & Society, 19*, 509–612.

Smith, B., & Sparkes, A. (2005). Men, sport, spinal cord injury and narratives of hope. *Social Science & Medicine, 61*, 1095–1105.

Smith, B., & Sparkes, A. (2008). Changing bodies, changing narratives and the consequences of tellability: A case study of becoming disabled through sport. *Sociology of Health and Illness, 30*, 217–236.

Smith, B., & Sparkes, A. (2009a). Narrative analysis and sport and exercise psychology: Understanding lives in diverse ways. *Psychology of Sport and Exercise, 10*, 279–288.

Smith, B., & Sparkes, A. (2009b). Narrative inquiry in sport and exercise psychology: What is it, and why might we do it? *Psychology of Sport and Exercise, 10*, 1–11.

Smith, B., & Sparkes, A. (2011). Multiple responses to a chaos narrative. *Health: An Interdisciplinary Journal for the Social Study of Health, Illness & Medicine, 15*, 38–53.

Smith, B., & Sparkes, A. C. (2002). Men, sport, spinal cord injury, and the construction of coherence: Narrative practice in action. *Qualitative Research, 2*, 143–171.

Sparkes, A. (2002). *Telling tales in sport and physical activity: A qualitative journey.* Champaign, IL: Human Kinetics Press.

Sparkes, A. (2005). Narrative analysis: Exploring the whats and the hows of personal stories. In M. Holloway (Ed.), *Qualitative research in health care* (pp. 91–209). Milton Keynes: Open University Press.

Sparkes, A., & Partington, S. (2003). Narrative practice and its potential contribution to sport psychology: The example of flow. *The Sport Psychologist, 17*, 292–317.

Sparkes, A., & Smith, B. (2002). Sport, spinal cord injuries, embodied masculinities, and narrative identity dilemmas. *Men and Masculinities, 4*, 258–285.

Sparkes, A., & Smith, B. (2003). Men, sport, spinal cord injury and narrative time. *Qualitative Research, 3*, 295–320.

Sparkes, A., & Smith, B. (2008). Men, spinal cord injury, memories, and the narrative performance of pain. *Disability & Society, 23*, 679–690.

Sparkes, A., & Smith, B. (2011). Inhabiting different bodies over time: Narrative and pedagogical challenges. *Sport, Education & Society, 16*, 357–370.

Sparkes, A., & Smith, B. (2012). Narrative analysis as an embodied engagement with the lives of others. In J. Holstein & J. Gubrium (Eds.), *Varieties of narrative analysis* (pp. 53–73). London: Sage.

Sparkes, A. & Smith, B. (forthcoming). *Qualitative research in sport, exercise & health sciences. From process to product.* London: Routledge.

Sparkes, A., Perez-Samaniego, V., & Smith, B. (2012). Social comparison processes, narrative mapping, and their shaping of the cancer experience: A case study of an elite athlete. *Health: An Interdisciplinary Journal for the Social Study of Health, Illness & Medicine, 16*(5), 467–488.

Squire, C. (2008). Experience-centered and culturally-orientated approaches to narrative. In M. Andrews, C. Squire & M. Tamboukou (Eds.), *Doing narrative research* (pp. 41–63). London: Sage.

Tilly, C. (2006). *Why?* Princeton, NJ: Princeton University Press.

Wendgraf, T. (2001). *Qualitative research interviewing: Biographic narrative and semi-structured methods.* London: Sage.

Wolcott, H. (1994). *Transforming qualitative data.* London: Sage.

CHAPTER 5

VISUAL METHODS IN PHYSICAL CULTURE: BODY CULTURE EXHIBITION

Emma Rich and Kerrie O'Connell

ABSTRACT

Purpose – *The purpose of the chapter is to introduce visual methods and, more specifically, arts-based forms of visual methods, as an innovative and emerging research approach within the study of sport and physical culture. The chapter examines the use of art and aesthetics as research data and as a representation issue. It draws upon the case of a research-based arts exhibition to represent and communicate research on bodies.*

Design/methodology/approach – *The chapter details an international collaborative research project exploring the impact of health policies and their imperatives on schools in the United Kingdom, Australia and New Zealand. The research formed the focus of an arts-based exhibition involving artists' interpretations of the authors' research findings. The chapter addresses salient epistemological and ontological issues of 'representation' and 'interpretation' in visual methods.*

Findings – *The chapter reveals how the use of arts-based approaches to research do not simply 'represent' research, but are constructive in the generation of new insights and forms of knowledge.*

Qualitative Research on Sport and Physical Culture
Research in the Sociology of Sport, Volume 6, 101–127
ISSN: 1476-2854/doi:10.1108/S1476-2854(2012)0000006008

Research limitations/implications – *The challenges of using arts-based and visual approaches to research are highlighted, particularly in terms of issues of knowledge interpretation. The ways in which these methods allow for lines of sight into life that written texts do not are highlighted.*

Originality/value – *The chapter provides an introduction to the use of arts-based visual methods in sport and physical culture research. Rather than focusing on visual methods solely as an approach to the collection of data, the chapter extends the discussion around visual methodology to include its use as a form of interpretation that generates and translates knowledge from a new perspective.*

Keywords: Visual methods; arts-based research; interpretation; research exhibitions

INTRODUCTION

In this chapter, we introduce the use of visual methods in research on physical culture as both a method of data collection and also as a way in which one might use visual material to construct and (re)present research findings. The use of photography, videos, artwork and other visual material as forms of data, or as an approach to assist in the collection of data, is now an established research approach. Extending the discussion around the notion of *the visual* in research, this chapter explores how the use of arts/aesthetics in research is both a data collection and a representation issue. By this, we mean that while visual methods are now well established as a means of data collection, they are also increasingly used to represent research findings in ways that go further than *empirically capturing* the data. Here, they may actually assist in the generation or translation of research from new perspectives. We outline how an arts-based approach was utilised in a large-scale international research project on how young people experience health policies and practices in schools focusing specifically on what can be described as new 'health imperatives' designed to tackled the emerging 'obesity epidemic'. Our project involved an exhibition where artists themselves were invited to interpret our research findings into aesthetic work. Drawing on examples from this exhibition, the chapter addresses some of the interpretive challenges one faces when translating via 'alternative' visual/aesthetic forms.

A BACKGROUND TO VISUAL METHODS

Before outlining the research exhibition in question and its link to visual methodologies, it is useful to explore how visual materials have, to date, been used within different research approaches within the field of physical cultural studies. For some time, qualitative research has been turning to 'visual culture' to better understand social and cultural meaning and context engaging with what is now recognised as a 'visual methodology' (Banks, 2007; Emmison & Smith, 2000; Margolis & Pauwels, 2011; Pink, 2007a, 2007b; Rose, 2007). There are a number of journals now dedicated to visual methods including *Visual Anthropology*, *Visual Studies* and *The Journal of Visual Culture*. Within this field of research, there is a great diversity in terms of theoretical and methodological approaches. Visual methods cover a wide range of empirical approaches including, but not limited to, ethnographic film (Loizos, 1992) photography and video (Cherrington & Watson, 2010), media analysis, social media, virtual methods and drawing (Gravestock, 2010), and Internet-based research (Miah & Rich, 2008). Thus, the particular 'case' reported in this chapter is merely one approach of many within visual research. It does not stand as representative of the entire field.

WHEN ARE VISUAL METHODS USED IN PHYSICAL CULTURAL STUDIES RESEARCH?

Over the last decade, there has been a rapid growth in the use of visual methods within sport and physical culture (SPC) research (Phoenix, 2010; Phoenix & Smith, 2011). In various fields and sub-disciplines such as the sociology of sport, physical cultural studies, pedagogy, physical education and sports psychology, visual methods are utilised as an innovative approach to undertake and represent research. Such was the growth of visual methods in these fields that the journal *Qualitative Research in Sport and Exercise* published a special edition, in 2010, on visual methods in physical culture research.

Given the extent to which physical culture is mediatised, it is not surprising that physical, cultural studies have turned to visual methodologies. Readers may choose to examine visual data to explore various dimensions of physical culture and the multiple meanings they might come to constitute in different contexts; indeed, one might argue that photography, art and cyberspace are just some of the many manifestations of broader physical culture. One of the longstanding questions regarding the specific value of these approaches is whether or not 'visual' forms may represent something that cannot be represented with words. Indeed, Phoenix (2010, p. 94) suggests that these visual forms allow us to ask different questions about physical culture such as: How are we *able* to see? How are we *allowed* to see? How are we *made* to see? *What* is being seen, and *how* is it socially shaped?

Visual approaches can provide a mechanism through which emotions, sensitive topics or lived experiences might be expressed more clearly than using linguistic text. For example, the use of photographic images created by the research participant, or indeed by the researcher, may assist in communicating particular embodied experiences, or emotions associated with such experiences. While these images may be utilised to document the evocative and/or the extreme, they are also important in conveying how mundane aspects of everyday life may yield significant insights into physical culture. For example, Hockey and Allen Collinson (2006), in their work on visual sociology and the distance runner's perspective, develop links between visual and auto-ethnographic data. Drawing together observation-based narratives and photographs in their attempt to outline subcultural knowledge and runners' 'ways of seeing', they use photographs to document runners' embodied feelings and experience of momentum en route. Elsewhere, Atkinson (2010, p. 118) using photo-elicitation 'infographically' illustrates the allure of 'post-sports' like fell running by using this technique to 'dig analytically deeper into existential experiences fell enthusiasts regularly described to me'. Drawing on Virilio and Petit (1999), Atkinson presents a series of pictures as a representational technique to capture the socially experienced body in fell running through visual symbols and icons. Cherrington and Watson (2010, p. 277) make similar observations of the potential for visual methods, in this case visual diaries, to 'deepen our engagement with the social world and encourage a richly textured account'. In this sense, visual methods may bring to life the social world in such a way as to invite a visceral relationship with physical cultural research.

While visual research involves not only the gathering and analysis of visual material, it also involves the *(re)presentation* of research *through* the visual. However, within the context of physical cultural studies, much less has been written about the dissemination and presentation of research through, for example arts-based approaches. Instead, visual research has traditionally been taken up through what Harrison (2002) distinguishes between the visual as *topic* and the visual as *resource*. The visual as topic might include visual media images and representations as the subject of analysis – such as an analysis of the media coverage of mega-events such as as resource = visual forms to explore a certain issue. (using image to understand exercise)

the Olympics. The visual as resource suggests the use of visual forms to explore a particular issue, for example the use of social media to examine how people construct meanings around exercise. The use of visual methods to collect data is perhaps the most utilised approach to the visual within existing research. This may involve the researcher working alongside the participant to co-produce visual material on a particular issue (Evans, Rich, Davies, & Allwood, 2008; Kluge, Grant, Friend, & Glick, 2010; Krane et al., 2010), such as through the method of 'photo-elicitation' (Harper, 2002).

In other studies, participants themselves may use cameras or other equipment to produce images and videos, which represent their experiences, meanings or emotions (Azzarito & Sterling, 2010; Sims-Gould, Clarke, Ashe, Naslund, & Liu-Ambrose, 2010). Azzarito and Sterling (2010), in their exploration of ways in which young people of different ethnicities in two urban schools engaged with physical culture in their everyday lives, asked participants to create a visual diary (called 'moving in my world') to represent their physicalities within various contexts. Similarly, Cherrington and Watson (2010) used video diaries as part of a sociological analysis of life, identity and the body for members of a university basketball team.

These approaches provide a means through which one can enter into the participants' world visually and challenge the traditionally hierarchical relationships inherent in academic research methods. Arts-based approaches have also been well used as a methodological approach to work with participants when addressing sensitive issues. For example, Evans et al. (2008), in their work on young anorexic women's experiences of health education and schools, encouraged the active involvement of the research participants in the generation of data (see Christensen & James, 2008; Oliver & Lalik, 2000). For many of these young women, the time during which they constructed their own visual posters about health education was a space in which they engaged with more critical dialogue about women's magazines and the constitution of bodily ideals. In addition, the themes emerging from the construction of posters and other arts-based material provided a useful way to approach such issues in interviews.

TRANSLATING AND REPRESENTING RESEARCH THROUGH ARTS-BASED APPROACHES

In this chapter, we discuss an additional aspect of the value of the visual in research on physical culture. This approach focuses on the utilisation of visual/arts-based forms to disseminate, (re)present and communicate research findings. We suggest that this approach enables researchers to pursue ways of interpreting and representing physical culture in more imaginative, and perhaps critical, ways. These arts-based interpretations of research issues can further understandings of, for example, the body, in ways which may differ from, yet also complement written narratives of, SPC.

Rather than being a process through which predetermined meanings are uniformly understood by the audience, the use of the visual provides an inter-discursive space through which social and cultural meanings around physical culture research can be negotiated, resisted and re-imagined. It is this space that provides a mechanism to construct new knowledge around particular research issues. In focusing on this aspect of visual representation and the dissemination of research, our discussion contributes to broader debates about the value of visual material throughout the entire research process within physical cultural studies. Indeed, Phoenix (2010) suggests there are three key aspects of debate about the use of visual methods in research on physical culture – these include interpretation, representation and ethics. In what follows, we outline a project based on artists' interpretations of the authors' work on body pedagogies (Rich, 2010; Rich & Evans, 2009) engaging with these aspects of the broader debates.

In this section, we outline a critical inquiry in terms of the use of an art exhibition to disseminate research undertaken by the author (Emma Rich) and colleagues (Evans et al., 2008; Rich, Evans, & De-Pian, 2011) exploring the ways young people constitute particular embodied subjectivities and learn about their health and their bodies through contemporary physical culture (learning both within and outside schools). In 2011, the authors, as researcher (Emma Rich) and artist/curator (Kerrie O'Connell), worked together to produce an art exhibition called 'Body Culture'.

Amid growing concerns about the rise in disordered eating and body dissatisfaction, this exhibition used a range of art forms to explore the impact of an increased focus on weighing, measuring and the surveillance on young people's bodies. The research informing this process was based on two large research projects: the first explored the 'schooling' experiences of young women with anorexia and the second explored the impact of new health imperatives on school policy and practice. Collectively, these research projects revealed how schools in many westernised societies have been expected, and even obliged, to respond to claims that their populations are in the midst of an 'obesity epidemic'. Many governments have charged schools and other state agencies with the responsibility for safeguarding young people's health by monitoring and regulating their weight, physical activity patterns and diets. Such concerns are driving what we describe as 'new health imperatives' – which prescribe the 'lifestyle' choices young people *should* make. The drive to tackle the putative 'obesity epidemic' has resulted in extensive government funding to support a number of health policies and school-based initiatives focused on the surveillance of young people's bodies and weight (e.g. annual weight checks, fingerprint screening in school canteens and removal of vending machines). In addition to this, various institutional, popular and cultural resources such as reality television, consumer culture, Internet-based tools and video gaming technologies focused on weight loss and body perfection provide new means through which young people come to understand their bodies, weight and social worth (Miah & Rich, 2008). What impact has this had on young people's eating, body image and sense of worth? What is the relationship between these forms of surveillance and the rise in disordered eating and body dissatisfaction? What does it mean to understand health as a simple matter of 'weight'? These critical questions were explored through the exhibition.

BODY CULTURE

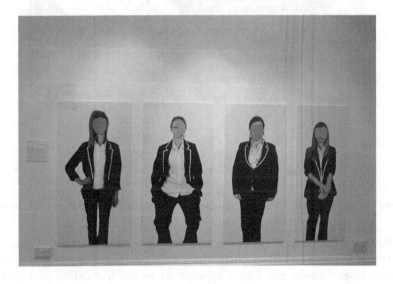

The Venus Effect. Photographic prints. Artist: Hester Jones (photography taken by Emma Rich).

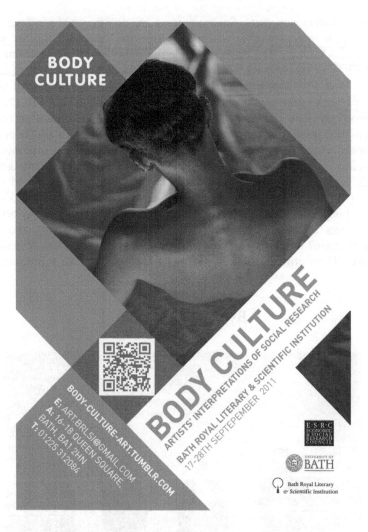

Body Culture Exhibition Poster. Designed by Rashpal Amrit and Kerrie O'Connell.

Research questions that engage with body practices and body regulation in this way lend themselves particularly well to arts-based research approaches. In particular, arts-based approaches to the translation of research perhaps realise the aspirations to develop more critical, affective and imaginative interpretations of physical culture. Readers might, of course, choose to undertake artwork themselves as researchers – indeed, many researchers now produce their own photography of other aesthetic forms to generate new insights. However, for the study outlined in this chapter, we adopted a research technique involving artists creating a range of aesthetic interpretations of our research findings.

Specifically, we commissioned 13 artists[1] to 'translate' our research into forms of performance art, conceptual sculptures, photography and other artistic forms. Each artist was given a series of published research papers (Evans, Rich, & Holroyd, 2004; Rich, 2006, 2010; Rich & Evans, 2005, 2009; Rich, Evans, & De-Pian, 2011) and asked to select a particular aspect of the work which inspired or interested them. These artists then underwent discussions with a museum curator and researcher about the construction of the art and its relationship with the research findings. This approach can be adopted with other research studies, where researchers can work with artists in the generation of new and creative forms of knowledge around the research. It is also useful to document this process for ethical and methodological reasons. We documented the process of interpretation through reflective diaries, informal discussion and interviews with the artists, focusing specifically on issues of representation, ethics and interpretation as critical debate. Readers might also focus specifically on how the aesthetic work changed understandings of the research phenomena through the new insights produced through aesthetic form that might not be produced through typically academic written form.

Art as Knowledge and the Artist as Inquirer

One of the benefits of drawing upon an arts-based approach to research is the extent to which it might allow one to develop a critical inquiry towards particular social issues. Working with artists may provide new ways through which to develop a critical approach: 'Art practice as research explores the capacity of visual research to create knowledge that can help us in understanding in a profound way the world we live in and how we learn to make sense of it' (Sullivan, 2010, p. xiii). As an artist and curator, Kerrie O'Connell's approach to practice involves running interdisciplinary art events to bring awareness of social science research and issues into the public domain. The creation of these events involves commissioning, facilitating, curating and working across art and social science contexts. As O'Connell (2012, p. 5) suggests:

> As an artist, I have always had a fascination with the living body and the relationship this has to science. My experience in making performance has been defined by my interest in the process of the body and the interventions of participants as part of this

process to create a work of art. As these interventions become situations, within a performance, the art process becomes the art. Out of this interest other questions have arisen, which has led me to think about performance as a form of action research.

This utilisation of visual forms to disseminate critical approaches and knowledge of the body therefore aligns with what is now recognised as 'public pedagogy':

[A] concept focusing on various forms, processes, and sites of education and learning occurring beyond formal schooling and is distinct from hidden and explicit curricula operating within and through school sites. (Sandlin, O'Malley, & Burdick, 2011; pp. 338–339)

In this sense, spaces such as art exhibitions become fruitful contexts in which to construct alternative pedagogies through which learning about a particular social issue might take place. In moving closer to a public pedagogical approach, we were cognizant of the value of art to potentially re-frame social science in a way that becomes meaningful:

To be real value in a public domain, the scientific knowledge has to be re-framed to engage audiences in terms specific to their culture and understanding, not in terms of those of the scientific community. (Russell, 2009, p. 5)

Those readers undertaking arts-based/visual research will face a series of seemingly practical questions, such as whether or not to display visual imagery with accompanying text. However, such questions connected to the ethical, methodological and paradigmatic position of the research. In our own project, there were some interesting discussion between artists, curator and researcher about the extent to which 'text' about the research and the artistic interpretation should accompany the visual performances and images exhibited. Like Newbury, as curator and researcher, our aspirations for the use of text and image/art were so that those experiencing the exhibition might be encouraged 'to switch back and forth between the images and the text, but the relationship is not one of pointing to what is *in* the image, rather it is an invitation for a more imaginative engage *with* the image and, by extension, the environment it represents' (Newbury, 2011, p. 656).

We interviewed the artists about their experiences of interpreting the research, and as one respondent commented:

I think that art is art and social research is another subject. It's good to connect them sometimes, but I think they should be understood independently. (Artist, exhibition)
I don't believe that art necessarily communicates research in the same way that a paper might, so may be unable to be more effective. I think that it gives a different perspective that may lead to further discussion around the topics of researched, but this is a difficult thing to control – and may not even be desired to be controlled. (Artist, exhibition)

Conversely, Pink (2007a, p. 66) points to the potential for 'continuities between the visual culture of an academic discipline and that of the subjects or collaborators in the research'. This continuity becomes even more pertinent given that we sought to undertake the research echoing the concerns of Saukko (2008, p. 77), 'in a hermeneutic feminist spirit' and felt a strong ethical duty to 'do justice' to those 'vulnerable' voices who have given their time and emotion within research (Saukko, 2008, p. 77). Harrison (2004, p. 132) captures some of these concerns well:

> It is not that pictures cannot tell stories in themselves, or that viewers cannot be invited to 'see' images in this way, but rather for the social scientist, we need to know what these stories or readings are ... It is for this reason that the possibility of visual narratives must encompass the idea that other forms of narration are essential to the realization of its context, its content and meaning. It's narration will provide us with an understanding of how it is such images do their 'work' as a material part of people's everyday lives. (2004, p. 132)

For readers hoping to engage artists with their research and publicly display/exhibit such work, one of the important methodological issues will thus be the extent to which interpretation of such work is left open or directed in some way by an accompanying narrative/text. Some of the artists expressed concerned that by placing text alongside the image, we may limit the opportunity for interpretation – what people may come to see, experience or know through their relationship with the image. Certainly, it was not our intention for the image to simplistically be 'treated as relatively transparent, allowing viewers access to what the re-searcher wants to show them' (Newbury, 2011, p. 654). While we do not seek to offer some sort of definitive position on this dilemma, it does prompt us to reflect critically on the nature of representation of research through the visual. In some forms, artists may indeed seek to align their visual representations as closely as possible to the conceptual aspects of research. For example, Stelios Manganis's sculpture (see Image 3) consists of ready-made objects arranged to present items used in 'measuring' the body. We asked Manganis to describe his interpretation of research:

> The research article has been a point of departure and a point of reference for the development of the proposed concept. The subject's body becomes simply another part in a closed circuit, in a complete mechanical assemblage. Body-monitoring systems translate corporeal information into data, relay this bodily data across information networks, and allow for the intervention of feedback mechanisms upon bodies. Since the body is part of this closed mechanical system, it cannot avoid being affected by this judgmental feedback, and thus becomes an instrument, a tool, or a machine at the disposal of consciousness, a vessel occupied by an animating, willful subjectivity. It has thus been my intention to create a closed system, a mechanism that would also involve

the visitor as one of its parts and which could affect this same visitor through the mechanism's 'feedback'. The surveillance would be superficial, yet overwhelming, and its feedback ought to be upfront and impersonally mechanical.

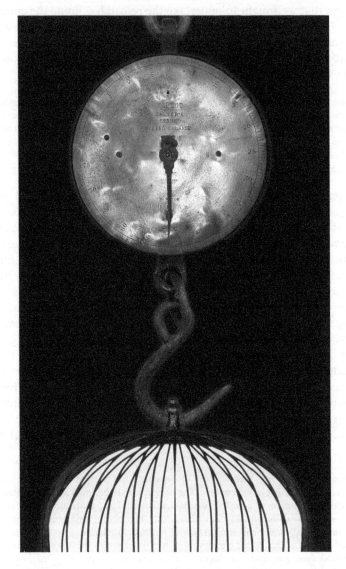

Stelios Manganis, *The Art of Sinking*, Sculpture – Metal, mirror, spring balance.

In our case example, we can thus see how consistency between purpose, paradigm and (re)presentation (and critical judgment of that representation) is crucial. Given the theoretical and methodological location of our research, we thus viewed the (re)presentation of the research through the exhibition not as a simple translation between a particular reality (research) and visual image/art, but rather involving the constitution of multiple realities at different moments. Each of these realities offers both new potentials for re-imagining social phenomena at the core of the research, while also posing ethical concerns about the duty to 'represent' the voices of those involved in the original research. Below, we explore the various ways in which these ontological possibilities emerged through the visual representation of the research.

Returning to our earlier methodological point, though, one can never guarantee that a particular reality might be read or interpreted in the way intended by the author/artist. In the context of visual imagery to assume that a sort of cause and effect relationship between intended representation of an image and actual interpretation would be to focus on 'how images affect bodies, that is to how pre-existent bodies are effected by pre-existent images' (Coleman, 2008, p. 164). To do so would be to reductively map research findings and visual representation onto an audience's 'reading' of that image, or as Coleman suggests, 'onto a prior distinction between subjects and objects' (2008, p. 164). Our interest instead is to avoid this distinction and explore the relational between particular bodies and between visual images and embodiment.

Artists' embodied experiences as sources of knowledge significantly shaped the layers of reality through which these visual images are produced:

> It was the direct quotes from young people that really stood out to me, the more I read the '*Obesity in Schools and Surveillance*' paper the more it struck me the language, the individual words that were jumping out, words like mechanism, monitoring, classification, collections, assemblages, reassembled, abstracted, protect and social control.
>
> There were a number of parts in the paper, '*Making Sense of Eating Disorders in Schools*' that really struck home for me. But there are two quotes in particular that I have just picked out ... they say a great deal. So, one of them was a young woman called Mia and she says, "I was bullied for being fat and then bullied for being thin ... I don't get it, how does that work?" For me, that's really powerful that statement, you can never win when you're a young woman; you're never perfect; you're neither one thing nor the other. That constant feeling that you're not achieving whatever this is goal is that you are supposed to reach and if you reach it, it is the wrong goal and the goalposts literally have changed. Another thing that really struck me creatively in terms of how I could start to visualise this piece of work was a young woman called Lydia who says, "I couldn't eat because when you have anorexia you can't. It's not that you don't want to, you just can't." Anorexia is like a person pulling you back from something. And for me that

really struck home in terms of someone being physically held up by this eating disorder. I guess that is partly where the idea came from of someone actually being restrained in a space by some sort of force that in a way contains some of this research.

The piece will consist of a female figure seen from behind straining to reach the top right hand corner of the frame. She is restrained by a 'rope' of text that extends from the bottom left hand corner of the frame. This 'rope' will be made up of direct quotes from Dr. Emma Rich's research documents relating to body surveillance in schools and the challenges posed to young women's sense of positive self-image. The intention is that the image will play with the viewer's sense of perspective, both literally and metaphorically, within that contained space. I envisage the room as stark, white and clinical but with the possible addition of a white board inscribed with a complex mathematical equation, referencing both the complexities of body surveillance and the link that many young people with eating disorders have with a sense of perfectionism. As well as making direct reference to Emma's research the work will also draw on Philip Gross's poem about his anorexic daughter, *The Wasting Game,* and the highly informative work by Kat Banyard, *The Equality Illusion.*

(Kamina Walton, artist).

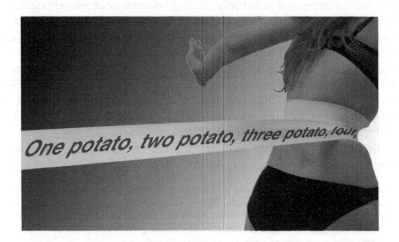

Kamina Walton. One potato, two potato ... Photographic print.

We drew upon Deleuze's (1992) perspective to consider how relationality thus impacts on what these young women's bodies might become in and through visual representation as they are reconstituted through the interpretations of those producing the image. The stories about these girls' bodies are re-imagined through the relationalities with the other bodies and embodied knowledge of those who 'represent' and 'interpret' them. Performance artist Alexandra Unger indicated how her own experience of her body is expressed through her performance: 'My interpretation is about the embodied experience, where my feelings of the body become the performance. I start from the subjective experience, and I aim to link that with other people'. The artist's inquiry in the *Body Culture* exhibition involves their own praxis art works, a combination of artistic intention and enquiry set in the parameters used in social science.

Pink (2007a, p. 175) suggests that visual methodologies 'evoke other people's sensory experience to an audience/reader' (Pink 2007a, p. 175). Such sensory experience is not only part of an audiences reaction to visual imagery, but is significant in promoting artists' to go beyond representing findings of a research paper and to undertake their own participatory action research. One artist reported that one of the most enjoyable aspects of the process was the way in which 'images immediately started to form in my head while reading the research'. For example, artist Samantha Sweeting experienced a sensory reaction to the experiences of the young women documented in the paper '*Anorexic Dis(connection)*' (Rich, 2006). Sweeting represented another person's diet for the course of a week as a piece of performance art in her interpretation of these issues. This dieting experience was presented visually through an exhibit of receipts, empty food packets and a reflective diary.

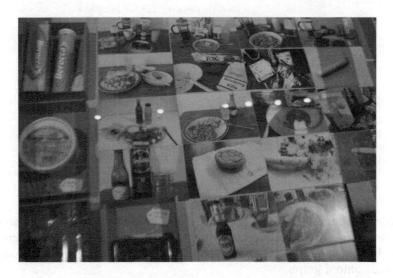

Samantha Sweeting. Food Diary. Documentation Study.

Wed 6th July

At SL - meetings all day + have to host
art handling workshop in gallery

Breakfast: - Glass of fresh orange juice + berocca
(Sheffield)   tablet
            - Special K Red Berry Cereal
            - 2 x black coffees

Lunch: - Small Vegetarian sushi selection
(St. Sheffield)   from Sainsburys
            - BBQ Thai flavoured crisps
            - Packet of Cadbury's Buttons
            - Bottle of Apple Beer

Snack: - Biscuit / cigarette

Dinner: - Tuna (in spring water) veg cous cous
              balsamic vinegar, rocket salad
            - 4 x crackers
            - Glass of water

            - 2 x Glühenfeldion + diet ginger ale
            - Cigarettes x 3

Samantha Sweeting. Food Diary. Documentation Study.

Similarly, Ciara McMahon, as part of her interpretation of 'Children's Bodies, Surveillance and the Obesity Crisis' (Rich et al., 2011) documented her hunger levels over four weeks and plotted these using embroidery threads onto a graph:

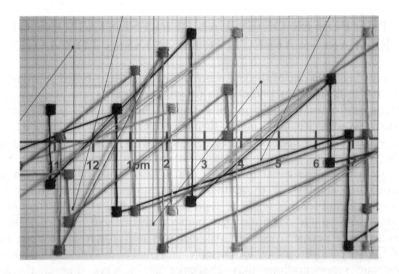

Ciara McMahon. Tangible Appetite. Plotted Graph, weeks 1–4. Paper and Embroidery Thread.

In their works, Sweeting and McMahon question the boundaries between an artist and a social science researcher. Artists are – like action researchers – spectators and self-reflectors; to understand knowledge often involves reflection and involvement of one's self and location in particular socio-economic, cultural and political context:

> The meanings of photographs are arbitrary and subjective; they depend on who is looking. The same photographic image may have a variety (perhaps conflicting) meanings invested in it at different stages of ethnographic research and representation, as it is viewed by different eyes and audiences in diverse temporal historical, spatial and cultural contexts. (Pink, 2007b, pp. 67–68)

Thus, as artists undertake a reflexive engagement with both the research and the subsequent art, it leads to both a self-renewal of knowledge and also a reconstitution of public pedagogy. The significant discussion with artists over this issue reflects an 'ongoing area of tension concerning the issue of representation appears to be the prioritising and valuing of verbal knowledge over visual knowledge' (Phoenix, 2010, p. 103).

THE POWER OF VISUAL REPRESENTATIONS OF RESEARCH: AFFECTIVE RESPONSES TO IMAGES

We now highlight one of the key benefits of using an arts-based approach to research in terms of its potential to provoke unique ways in which people 'interact' with, understand and utilise research findings. Arts-based research translation may provide a means through which to re-frame knowledge in ways that engage a broader audience, or indeed an audience that might not otherwise respond to our research. What kinds of research issues in SPC research might this assist in developing? These forms of translation are particularly helpful for those undertaking studies using a critical and interpretive approach. Aesthetic representations may provoke emotional, creative and unique responses that enable individuals to experience things through new perspectives. Such perspectives may foster more open and positive ways of perceiving, for example, marginal body types or disabilities. Aesthetic representations may challenge us in ways that create new sensitivities towards particular aspects of SPC. Readers might then want to ask if the artistic and creative process of translating research might be more effective in transforming processes, views or meanings which are deemed to be problematic. In what follows below, we outline how these 'responses' are cultivated through a focus on *affect*.

In the process of re-framing knowledge to engage audiences, through visual means, we suggest that 'affect' is a significant aspect of the ways in which audiences respond to images. As Probyn (2004, p. 26) suggests, 'affect amplification makes us care about things'. In focusing on relationalities and affect, we are thus able to better understand the role of visual material not only in terms of what they might *mean* but also what an image *does* as one experiences a different relationality with it. Focusing on the affect of these images 'means that we can distinguish the intensity of an image, its affective potential, from its content' (Featherstone, 2010, p. 209). It is the intensity of these images (e.g. the physical manipulation of flesh) and its affectivity (rather than the mere representation and interpretation of meaning), which underscores the potential for visual representations and the types of realities they imply about particular aspects of physical culture (in this case the body and health).

This discussion is perhaps best explicated through an example of one of the performance pieces included in the *Body Culture* exhibition. Within the research papers presented to the artists, a significant finding was the tendency for many of the young people in our research to associate 'fat' with the 'abject' (Kristeva, 1982) – or, 'bodily fluids, people, objects and places that are regarded as unclean, impure and even immoral' (Kenway & Bullen, 2009, p. 163). As echoed in the words of, Milly, one of our Year 7 participants:

> I think that it shows that someone's measuring themselves and they're quite concerned and it's *just disgusting a little* bit ... yeah and it's overflowing ... I think if you want to like make people stop it, because some people find it really hard and like you can't do it, but if you want to make them stop, I think you should show 'em really scary stories because that's what made me think. Because you look at it and you think 'oh my God'.

But how might one convey or disseminate this visually? Cited in Zembylas (2007), Gatens (1996, p. 169) remind us of the potential of the performing body to produce particular e/affects through its relationality with other bodies:

> Bodies of all sorts are in constant relation with other bodies; some of these relations are compatible and give rise to joyful affects which may in turn increase the intensive capacity of a body; others are incompatible relations and which give rise to sad or debilitating affects which at their worst may entirely create a body's integrity. (Gatens, 1996, p. 169, cited in Zembylas, 2007)

Affects are not simply emotional responses, or selective reactions, but rather 'what constitutes an affective response is hugely complex, and is in part the result of an embodied history to which and with which the body reacts, including how the classroom [and fatness] is conceived and practiced' (Probyn, 2004, p. 30). Thus, an artist's embodied history is crucial in the construction of a particular art form, representing a sort of intensity of reaction to various voices, experiences and findings evident within the research papers. Equally, the potential for affect through visual imagery is precisely what 'opens up' the possibility for capturing that which potentially cannot be wholly articulated (or made more accessible) through words. In Alexandra Unger's performance at the Body Culture exhibition, she engaged purposefully with the 'abject' in a way in which could perhaps not produce the same reactions through words alone:

> I would like to do a performance, which has the provisional title, 'Fantasy to Let Go' in which I will allow myself to lose control and to be seen losing the control. I will interact with a block of gelatin, destroy its square shape, eat it but also soil myself, and the floor around me. The sound of handled gelatin tends to be repulsive. I would like this eventually to turn into a sensual experience, where I am making peace with food and body, connecting the outside with the inside of it and make peace with this connection.

When attending this performance on the opening night of the exhibition, the affective qualities of this performance were clear; many of the audience members found aspects of the performance 'disgusting' and/or reacted physical with what Probyn (2004, p. 29) calls the 'goose bump effect; that moment when a text sets off a frisson of feelings, remembrances, thoughts, and the bodily actions that accompany them'. Elsewhere, Featherstone

(2010, p. 200) observes: 'It is an unstructured non-conscious experience transmitted between bodies, which have the capacity to create affective resonances below the threshold of articulated meaning'. Often, members of the audience were unable to give any precise justification for why these images prompted feelings of intense disgust; it was just something produced/ experienced in relation to the loss of control, fluids and food products smeared over the body. This had powerful generative intensities in the formation of people's relation with the aspect of physical culture being explored. In Featherstone's (2010) work on affect, body and image, he suggests that this points towards the affective body – a 'body without an image' which comes to shape encounters such as those described above, in complex ways. As the artist Alexandra Unger explains about her performance:

> I always start from myself or from another person, but I always start from the subjective experience and I aim to link the personal experience to other people's experience. For this exhibition, I linked my piece with a text called, 'Managing Anorexia as an Illness and Identity'. In this text, there is a piece about how anorexics burn calories by wearing little clothes, so that they burn more, or if they have to take something out of the wardrobe, they will pick one thing at a time and go back and forth several times … so in a way they control constantly their body. So my piece has a first part, which is about control, but what I really wanted to do was lose control so that's the main point of my performance: to lose control.

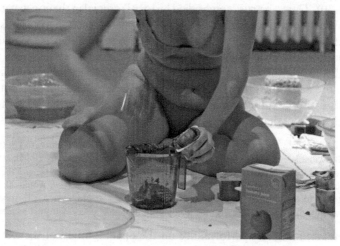

Alexandra Unger. Fantasy to let go. Live Performance.

The assertion that visual performances can articulate something that might not be articulated verbally was particularly striking as we worked with colleagues to think about the more recent developments in academic understandings of the body. Clearly, the manner in which young people respond to expectations and pressures associated with body norms and health imperatives obviously vary, and the sociology of education has been adept at revealing how the culture of school is mediated and sometimes opposed by some young people. A number of the artworks in the exhibition offered powerful representations of surveillance, such as the piece by Hannah Gardener:

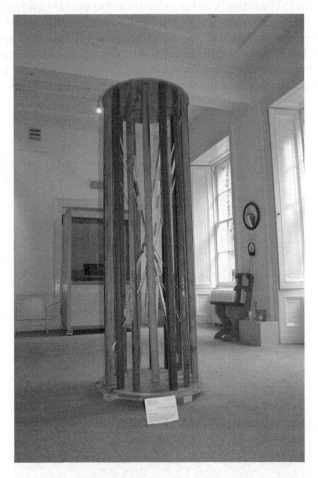

Hannah Gardener. The Surveillance Assemblage. Sculpture. Reclaimed wood and tape measures.

Readers might wish to consider exploring the reactions of particular audiences to their aesthetic works. This may be particularly beneficial if there are critical groups that the research seeks to engage with or wishes to challenge inequalities. During the exhibition, we undertook body image workshops with children and young people from local schools, engaging with the artwork and discussing their own views about body culture and body image. During the course of these workshops, we found young people developed a more critical engagement with body perfection ideals and current health policies. The artwork at the exhibition thus enabled an approach that allowed for critical transformative knowledge to be developed in ways which narrative/written representations, or indeed other pedagogical approaches, might not have enabled. The creative medium provides a degree of freedom which enables the artist and research to more intimately (re)present through intensified examinations of bodily practices and cultures.

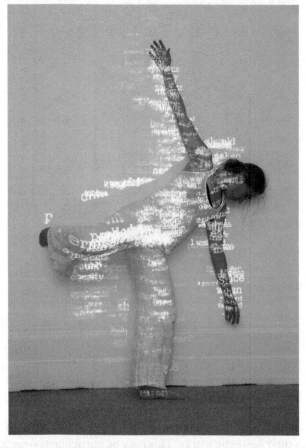

Performer Marina Tsartsara. Collaboration with visual Artist Jeremy Radvan. Ever Changing. Live Performance.

CONCLUSION

While the use of visual methods as a source of data or as a tool to collect data is now well recognised within the field of physical cultural studies, less has been written about the use of visual mediums to disseminate research through 'art practice' or 'visual scholarship' (Newbury, 2011). We suggest that arts-based methods as part of the larger research process draw on particular creative sensibilities and forms of communication to produce particular insights that conventional written text might not. In this sense, arts-based methods are different than more traditional approaches, but this does not mean that they should replace them outright. Visual interpretations in this sense may offer an affective dimension to the interpretation of physical culture in a way that cannot be articulated and/or accessed through words alone.

Certainly, emerging innovations in scholarship are already on our horizon through the bringing together of artists and scholars to address significant research issues. For example, Miah's (2008) creative text, *Human Futures*, brings together leading intellectuals, artist and even science fictions writers to interrogate the future of humanity, producing an illuminating insight into contested bodies and encounters with the future. Texts like these bring visual scholarship to new audiences and through provocation, artistic interpretation present new manifestations not only of research but also of our cultural imagination.

Equally, in this chapter we have tried to document the process of engaging with artists in a process of interpreting and representing a volume of research focusing on body culture and pedagogy. Far from being a simple representation of research findings, through visual methods, physical culture can be re-imagined in ways that invite affective responses and may help us to attend to public pedagogy agendas. For instance, they might encourage others to work with and 'acknowledge and work with the affective reaction' (Probyn, 2004, p. 30) they have to particular bodies – including images circulating within popular culture, actual bodies in schools and also bodies which may circulate as a sort of invisible but pervasive presence.

Having undertaken research that draws on arts-based methodology, its benefits and challenges are multiple. Artistic expression and interpretation can be deeply personal. The particular medium and artistic form may be meaningful to some but not all. Readers must navigate an array of methodological challenges if they are to consider translating their research findings into visual/artistic form. For example, some members of the audience at our exhibition found particular artworks too abstract and thus without meaning. For others, the affective and aesthetic elements of the

[handwritten margin note:] affective, but should not replace well research – not replace

artwork, even if 'abstract', prompted an emotional reaction that brought them to new perspectives on the body and schooling. In their research studies, readers should consider what judgement criteria might be used in relation to these arts-based (re)presentations of their research. Importantly, there should be a clear connection between the paradigmatic approach and the purpose of the exhibition.

When designing an arts-based research approach, it is therefore important to consider a range of questions – the extent to which the aesthetic dimension might enhance an understanding of physical culture, whether you will undertake the artistic (re)presentation yourself or with through the work of an 'artist', or the extend to which you will direct the interpretation of the research both in relation to the artist and the audience. Given all of this, it might not be surprising that this research approach is not as 'linear' as others. Arts/visual-based inquiries and (re)presentations of research studies may provide a way of knowing which does not seek to replace other (re)presentations or interpretations of research, but which complements them and may provide a more complete way of understanding or challenging particular meanings and practices within physical culture. One of the benefits of (re)presenting research in this way is that it may generate new insights which might not be possible through narrative/written text. As audiences develop embodied/affective sensibilities through their engagement with artworks, the critical 'translational' properties of research may be enhanced. Equally, readers might want to explore these embodied sensibilities that temper individuals' reactions to particular 'research issues' as some indication of embodied and deeply embedded meanings within physical cultures.

FIVE KEY READINGS

1. Banks, M. (2007). *Using visual data in qualitative research.* **London: Sage.**
This book is helpful for exploring the range of ways in which visual images might be used in research.

2. Phoenix, C. (2010). Seeing the world of physical culture: The potential of visual methods for qualitative research in sport and exercise. *Qualitative Research in Sport and Exercise, 2*(2) 93–108.
This paper gives an overview of how visual methods are currently used within the research on physical culture and explores issues of interpretation and representation.

3. Pink, S. (2007a). *Doing visual ethnography* **(2nd ed.). London: Sage.**
This is an essential text for exploring the theoretical, methodological and ethical issues confronting those using visual methods approaches.

4. Rose, G. (2007). *Visual methodologies: An introduction to the interpretation of visual materials.* **London: Sage.**
Rather than focusing on the visual to collect data, this book examines how to 'read' visual material that is already present in culture. This is useful for those researching visual aspects of physical culture.

5. McNiff, S. (2008). Art-based research. In J. G. Knowles & A. L. Cole (Eds.) *Handbook of the arts in qualitative research: Perspectives, methodologies, examples, and issues* **(Chapter 3, pp. 29–40). London: Sage.**
A useful text for those hoping to utilise art as a practice of enquiry or through which to disseminate research knowledge.

NOTE

1. **Annabelle Craven Jones:** http://www.annabellecravenjones.wordpress.com
   Ana Mendes: http://www.anamendes.com
   Alexandra Unger: http://www.alexandraunger.com
   Ciara McMahon: http://www.livinggift.ie/leaky-self/blog
   Hannah Gardiner: http://hannahgardiner.co.uk/
   Hester Jones: http://www.hesterjones.com
   Kamina Walton: http://www.kaminawalton.co.uk
   Kirsten Linning: http://www.linning.co.uk
   Marina Tsartsara: http://www.marinatsartsara.co.uk
   Sally Lemsford: http://www.45poundsplus.co.uk
   Samantha Sweeting: http://www.samanthasweeting.com
   Sarah Lüdemann: http://www.sarahluedemann.com
   Stelios Manganis: http://www.steliosmanganis.com

REFERENCES

Atkinson, M. (2010). Fell running in post-sport territories. *Qualitative Research in Sport and Exercise, 2*(2), 109–132.

Azzarito, L., & Sterling, J. (2010). 'What it was in my eyes': Picturing youths' embodiment in 'real' spaces. *Qualitative Research in Sport and Exercise, 2*(2), 209–228.

Banks, M. (2007). *Using visual data in qualitative research.* London: Sage.

Cherrington, J., & Watson, B. (2010). Shooting a diary, not just a hoop: Using video diaries to explore the embodied everyday contexts of a university basketball team. *Qualitative Research in Sport and Exercise, 2*(2), 267–281.

Christensen, P., & James, A. (2008). *Research with children: Perspectives and practices.* Abingdon, UK: Routledge.

Coleman, R. (2008). The becoming of bodies. *Feminist Media Studies, 8*(2), 163–179.

Deleuze, G. (1992). Ethology: Spinoza and us. In J. Crary & S. Kwinter (Eds.), *Incorporations* (pp. 625–633). New York: Zone.

Emmison, M., & Smith, P. (2000). *Researching the visual: Images, objects, contexts and interactions in social and cultural inquiry.* London: Sage.

Evans, J., Rich, E., Davies, B., & Allwood, R. (2008). *Education, disordered eating and obesity discourse: Fat fabrications.* Oxon, UK: Routledge.

Evans, J., Rich, E., & Holroyd, R. (2004). Disordered eating and disordered schooling: What schools do to middle class girls. *British Journal of Sociology of Education, 25*(2), 123–142.

Featherstone, M. (2010). Body, image and affect in consumer culture. *Body and Society, 16*(1), 193–221.

Gatens, M. (1996). Through a spinozist lens: Ethology, difference, power. In P. Patton (Ed.), *Deleuze: A critical reader* (pp. 162–187). Oxford, UK: Blackwell.

Gravestock, H. (2010). Embodying understanding: Drawing as research in sport and exercise. *Qualitative Research in Sport and Exercise, 2*(2), 196–208.

Harper, D. (2002). Talking about pictures: A case for photo elicitation. *Visual Studies, 17*(1), 13–26.

Harrison, B. (2002). Seeing health and illness worlds – Using visual methodologies in a sociology of health and illness: A methodological review. *Sociology of Health and Illness, 24*(6), 856–872.

Harrison, B. (2004). Photographic visions and narrative inquiry with commentaries and response to Poddiakov, Chalfen and rich. In M. Bamberg & M. Andrews (Eds.), *Considering counter-narratives: Narrating resisting and making sense* (pp. 113–136). Amsterdam, The Netherlands: John Benjamins.

Hockey, J., & Allen Collinson, J. (2006). Seeing the way: Visual sociology and the distance runner's perspective. *Visual Studies, 21*(1), 70–81.

Kenway, J., & Bullen, E. (2009). Consuming skin: Dermographies of female subjection and abjection. In J. Sandlin & P. McLaren (Eds.), *Living and learning in the shadow of the "Shopocalypse": Towards a critical pedagogy of consumption* (pp. 157–168). New York: Routledge.

Kluge, M. L., Grant, B. C., Friend, L., & Glick, L. (2010). Seeing is believing: Telling the 'inside' story of a beginning masters athlete through film. *Qualitative Research in Sport and Exercise, 2*(2), 282–292.

Krane, V., Sally, R., Ross, S. R., Miller, M., Rowse, J. L., Ganoe, K., … Lucas, C. B. (2010). Power and focus: Self-representation of female college athletes. *Qualitative Research in Sport and Exercise, 2*(2), 175–195.

Kristeva, J. (1982). *Powers of horror: An essay on abjection (L.S. Roudiez, trans.).* New York: Columbia University Press.

Loizos, P. (1992). *Innovation in ethnographic film.* Manchester, UK: Manchester University Press.

Margolis, E., & Pauwels, L. (2011). *The Sage handbook of visual research methods.* London: Sage.

Miah, A. (2008). *Human futures: Art in an age of uncertainty.* Liverpool, UK: Liverpool University Press.

Miah, A., & Rich, E. (2008). *The medicalization of cyberspace.* Oxon, UK: Routledge.

Newbury, D. (2011). Making arguments with images: Visual scholarship and academic publishing. In E. Margolis & L. Pauwels (Eds.), *Handbook of visual research methods* (pp. 651–664). London: Sage.

O'Connell, K. (2012). *Publicising qualitative research communication and cross-pollination of social science.* Unpublished dissertation.

Oliver, K. L., & Lalik, R. (2000). *Bodily knowledge: Learning about equity & justice with adolescent girls.* Oxford, UK: Peter Lang.

Phoenix, C. (2010). Seeing the world of physical culture: The potential of visual methods for qualitative research in sport and exercise. *Qualitative Research in Sport and Exercise, 2*(2), 93–108.

Phoenix, C., & Smith, B. M. (Eds.). (2011). *The world of physical culture in sport and exercise: Visual methods for qualitative research.* Abingdon, UK: Routledge.

Pink, S. (2007a). *Doing visual ethnography* (2nd ed.). London: Sage.

Pink, S. (2007b). Walking with video. *Visual Studies, 22*(3), 240–252.

Probyn, E. (2004). Teaching bodies: Affects in the classroom. *Body & Society, 10*(4), 21–43.

Rich, E. (2006). Anorexic (Dis)connection: Managing anorexia as an illness and an identity. *Sociology of Health and Illness, 28*(3), 284–305.

Rich, E. (2010). Obesity assemblages and surveillance in schools. *International Journal of Qualitative Studies in Education, 23*(7), 803–821.

Rich, E., & Evans, J. (2005). Making sense of eating disorders in schools. *Discourse: Studies in the Cultural Politics of Education, 26*(2), 247–262.

Rich, E., & Evans, J. (2009). Now I am NO-body, see me for who I am: The paradox of performativity. *Gender and Education, 21*(1), 1–16.

Rich, E., Evans, J., & De-Pian, L. (2011). Childrens' bodies, surveillance and the obesity crisis. In E. Rich, L. F. Monaghan & L. Aphramor (Eds.), *Debating obesity: Critical perspectives.* London: Palgrave.

Rose, G. (2007). *Visual methodologies: An introduction to the interpretation of visual materials.* London: Sage.

Russell, N. (2009). *Communicating science: Professional, popular, literary.* Cambridge, UK: Cambridge University Press.

Sandlin, J. A., O'Malley, M. P., & Burdick, J. (2011). Mapping the complexity of public pedagogy scholarship: 1894–2010. *Review of Educational Research, 81*, 338–375.

Saukko, P. (2008). *The anorexic self: A personal, political analysis of a diagnostic discourse.* Albany, NY: SUNY Press.

Sims-Gould, J., Clarke, L. H., Ashe, M. C., Naslund, J., & Liu-Ambrose, T. (2010). Renewal, strength and commitment to self and others: Older women's reflections of the benefits of exercise using Photovoice. *Qualitative Research in Sport and Exercise, 2*(2), 250–266.

Sullivan, G. (2010). *Art practice as research.* London: Sage.

Virilio, P., & Petit, P. (1999). *Politics of the very worst.* New York: Semiotext(e).

Zembylas, M. (2007). The specters of bodies and affects in the classroom: A rhizo-ethological approach. *Pedagogy, Name: Culture & Society, 15*(1), 19–35.

CHAPTER 6

MEDIA ANALYSIS IN PHYSICAL CULTURAL STUDIES: FROM PRODUCTION TO RECEPTION

Brad Millington and Brian Wilson

ABSTRACT

Purpose – *To discuss the history and relevance of audience research as it pertains to sport and physical culture and to demonstrate an approach to doing audience research.*

Design/methodology/approach – *A step-by-step overview of a study conducted by the authors is provided. The study examined ways that groups of young males in a Vancouver, Canada, high school interpreted images of masculinity in popular media, and ways these same youth performed masculinity in physical education classes. We reflect on how studying interpretations (using focus groups) and lived experiences (using participant observation and in-depth interviews) in an integrated fashion was helpful for understanding the role of media in the everyday lives of these youth. We also describe how the hegemony concept guided our data interpretation.*

Findings – *We highlight how, on the one hand, the young males were critical of media portrayals of hegemonic forms of masculinity and, on the other hand, how these same males attempted to conform to*

Qualitative Research on Sport and Physical Culture
Research in the Sociology of Sport, Volume 6, 129–150
Copyright © 2012 by Emerald Group Publishing Limited
All rights of reproduction in any form reserved
ISSN: 1476-2854/doi:10.1108/S1476-2854(2012)0000006009

norms associated with hegemonic masculinity in physical education classes. We emphasise that our multi-method approach was essential in allowing us to detect the incongruity between youth 'interpretations' and 'performances'.

Research limitations/implications – *Limitations of audience research are discussed, and the epistemological underpinnings of our study are highlighted.*

Originality/value – *The need for audience research in physical cultural studies is emphasised. We suggest that researchers too often make claims about media impacts without actually talking to audiences, or looking at what audiences 'do' with information they glean from media.*

Keywords: Audience; media; sport; masculinity; physical education

INTRODUCTION

The 1999 film *Man on the Moon* depicts a notable exchange between Andy Kaufman (played by Jim Carey), the eccentric, satirical comedian, and the talent agent George Shapiro (played by Danny DeVito). After an appearance on the Merv Griffin show in which Andy, in the style of a professional wrestler, shamelessly disparaged Griffin's female audience, then fought out a live wrestling match with a female volunteer, George frets over Andy's waning popularity. 'Andy, they detest you', George says, 'the next time you make an appearance, women are gonna picket', Andy's response – 'You think so?' – is met with further insistence from George: "Yes! Because you have not given them any clues that this is a parody' (Forman, 1999).

Andy's comical wrestling outfit notwithstanding, George is right to express concern over how audiences will make sense of Andy's lampooning of masculinity and wrestling culture. Indeed, the question of how people interpret media 'texts' – whether they be TV shows, films, radio programmes, magazines, or other communication materials – has long been of interest to researchers and cultural commentators. This includes scholars studying sport and physical culture (SPC), who have made contributions over time to the field of media analysis commonly referred to as 'audience research' or 'reception studies'. And while much has been learned over the years about the meanings people extract from the media texts they encounter, researchers also tend to agree with George that the views of media audiences can never be guaranteed in advance.

In this chapter, we explore the rich and nuanced tradition of audience research and consider its relationship with SPC. In doing so, we highlight the influential work on audiences by cultural studies pioneers like Stuart Hall and David Morley, describe key methodological and theoretical developments in the field and examine the (still limited) role of 'the audience' in SPC work to date. Finally, and with the goal of illuminating the methods and theories that oftentimes underlie audience research, we describe a study we conducted with a group of young male media consumers in Vancouver, Canada. The study was designed to help us understand how the teenagers we studied interpret 'hegemonic' portrayals of masculinity in popular culture, and then (as is characteristic of more recent reception studies) consider these interpretations in relation to our research participants' experiences and actions in other parts of their lives (physical education [PE] class in particular). Along the way, we highlight the benefits that accompany this type of media analysis, while offering reflections on the challenges we faced as well.

Audience Research in Context: Studying Production and Representation

As noted above, the tradition of audience research conducted by scholars studying SPC is embedded in a much larger field of media studies – a field that includes research on media production and media 'texts'. Studies of mass or mainstream media production – which we distinguish here from alternative media production, like personal blogs – tend to be concerned with the processes and power relations underlying the creation of, for example, newspaper articles, television programmes or major corporate-driven websites of all kinds. 'Processes' here often refers to components of media production like editing, graphical design, commentating, photography and other technical skills that come together to form an 'invisible apparatus of presentation' ('invisible' because it is unseen by the viewer – Clarke & Clarke, 1982; c.f. Silk, 1999). 'Power relations', meanwhile, refers to the fact that media production is never a neutral process; rather, producers 'encode' media in ways that tend to (intentionally or inadvertently) privilege a particular set of ideas and, in turn, implicitly or explicitly delegitimise (i.e. call into question) others. In this sense, mass media contents can be seen as socially constructed, emerging from the biases that inform the development of editorial practices and the (often corporate-influenced) structures that shape how texts are produced.

Key studies of sport media production demonstrate this crucial link between the formation of mass media and the legitimising of cultural knowledge (e.g. Darnell & Sparks, 2005; Millington, 2009; Scherer & Jackson, 2008; Silk, 1999). One of the most frequently cited projects of this kind is MacNeill's (1996) ethnographic study of the Canadian Television Network's (CTV) coverage of men's hockey at the 1988 Calgary Olympics. Through interviews with various members of CTV's production team, and through her own observations of production 'in process' (for instance work routines, technology usage, relations between producers and so forth), MacNeill developed a keen understanding of how coverage of hockey games is far from an exercise in unbiased storytelling. Rather, MacNeill showed how CTV legitimised a narrative of Canada's unassailable 'ownership' of hockey, despite a 30-plus-year interregnum since the country's last gold medal in the sport. Indeed, the broadcast crew saw hockey as Canada's 'natural' possession, since Canadians (and, more precisely, Canadian men) were thought to embody the game's rough and tumble spirit. This mentality in turn affected actual production practices – for instance, it foretold a preference for tight camera angles that highlighted personal acumen and grit, rather than the overall flow of the game. In this sense, then, MacNeill's research usefully demonstrates how select (rather than impartial) ideas are foregrounded in media, as CTV was shown to craft a narrative that emphasised certain themes (Canadian nationalism; a view of hockey as a game 'for men' who are gritty and tough) over others.

And yet, despite the intentions of media producers, once a media text is produced and published, it is then open to interpretation. A second form of media analysis involves the study of finalised texts themselves – or what is commonly referred to as 'textual' analysis – with an eye on the meanings they convey (intentionally or not). For this style of research, the 'audience' is the researcher who chooses to analyse the media text, although most researchers offer hints or ideas about how they think other audiences (like those targeted by the producers of the text) might be influenced by the text in the end.

Researchers have adopted a range of strategies for studying media texts. Sometimes they are interested simply in identifying 'how often' a particular term or theme is written, shown or spoken – for example, how often female athletes are covered in news media in relation to male athletes. This quantitative form of textual analysis is called 'content analysis'. More commonly, however, researchers strive to qualitatively analyse the meanings connoted by SPC media, usually by considering:

- Precisely what is said or shown in the text (e.g. whether female athletes are written or talked about for their athletic achievements or their physical appearance). This is sometimes known as the 'denotative' or surface level of analysis.
- How the meaning of the text is influenced by and reinforced through its relationship with other texts (e.g. images of females in other sport media) – what is sometimes known as 'intertextuality'.
- The broader contexts in which the text exists, and how these contexts might give deeper meaning to the text (at the 'connotative' level). For example, scholars who study female athlete portrayals often suggest that the texts they study are best understood in relation to: the historical exclusion of girls and women from sport; the tendency for social changes that favour female participation in sport to be accompanied by changes that undermine these progressions (e.g. more participants and funding accompanied by fewer administrative jobs for women) or sweatshop employment for women in countries of the Global South in factories that produce athletic apparel that is consumed by wealthier women of the Global North.

Variations exist within this qualitative form of textual analysis, often based on one's theoretical approach (e.g. there are varying forms of 'discourse analysis' – see Markula & Silk, 2011). Nonetheless, those engaging in textual analysis of SPC are commonly interested in power relations, and generally share an assumption that media texts have the capacity to make certain ideas appear 'right' or commonsensical.

Within the impressive catalogue of textual analyses of SPC media, Messner, Dunbar, and Hunt's (2000) study on the 'Televised Sports Manhood Formula' is one we found especially influential for our own research. At the outset of their study, Messner and his colleagues were interested in the messages contained in televised sports programming known to be popular among young males. They thus began their research by selecting a specific sample of texts for analysis: for example, two broadcasts of the sports highlight programme *SportsCenter*, two professional wrestling broadcasts, two broadcasts of the American show *Monday Night Football* and so forth. They then combined quantitative (content) and qualitative (textual) forms of analysis, first identifying key themes and the frequency with which they emerged (e.g. the valorising of violence), and second by unearthing the precise ways these themes were legitimised (e.g. the description of those eschewing violence as 'soft'). In total, Messner, Dunbar, and Hunt suggest there is a 'formula' at work in sports media that serves to normalise the idea that the 'ideal' male is tough, aggressive, overtly heterosexual and a 'winner' in a 'Man's World' (p. 390). They then connect these findings to broader cultural trends, suggesting that the normalising of this type of masculinity helps explain 'why so many boys and men continue to take seemingly irrational risks, submitting to pain and injury, and risk long-term debility or even death by playing hurt' (p. 392).

The Audience Research Tradition

What cannot be known from production studies, and furthermore what is difficult to surmise from textual analyses, are the various ways that audiences make sense of the media they are watching, reading and/or hearing. As Messner and his colleagues (2000) acknowledge:

> It is not possible, based merely on our textual analysis of sports programs, to explicate precisely what kind of impact these shows, and the Televised Sports Manhood Formula, have on their young male audiences. That sort of question is best approached through direct research with audiences. (p. 392)

Fortunately, there is also an impressive tradition of reception studies from which researchers facing this type of conundrum can draw.

Perhaps the most significant contribution to the practice of studying media audiences came with the publication of Stuart Hall's (1980 [1973]) brief synopsis of media 'Encoding/Decoding'. It is true that before the release of this essay, there was a significant body of literature on media consumers, with a particular focus on TV audiences. But Hall felt this work was – in his words – 'dogged' by a deterministic understanding of audience habits. That is to say, researchers commonly took interest in media 'effects', and in doing so assumed that (a) media messages were understood exactly as intended and (b), more broadly, that audience members were inherently passive. By contrast, Hall theorised that there were no 'guarantees' in how (for example) a TV show would be 'decoded', since audiences were in fact *active* in their relationships with media. Consumers might well take away a 'hegemonic' interpretation of a text (i.e. one perfectly in line with the producers' intentions), yet they might also take away a critical, 'oppositional' view, or a 'negotiated' one that accepts some of the producer's ideas and rejects others. This variability in media consumption stemmed, in Hall's view, from the diversity of media audiences themselves; just as the CTV crew in MacNeill's study approached the *production* of media with their own biases, so too do audiences approach *consumption* with differing political views (or what Hall called 'frameworks of knowledge') that are potentially influenced by their differing social positions (e.g. varying class backgrounds).

Hall acknowledged that his theorising of media 'decoding' needed to be tested empirically – which is to say, research was needed that actually gauged audience perceptions. Following Hall's lead, interest in media audiences flourished through the 1980s, with scholars using methods examined elsewhere in this book – for example, interviews and focus groups – to unearth patterns of media reception among different audience groups. Morley (1980), for example, put Hall's conjectures to work, investigating how 26 audience groups from different backgrounds and occupations understood the British news programme *Nationwide*. And while Morley found it difficult to surmise that one's social position (e.g. race and class) necessarily influenced her or his decoding of *Nationwide*, he nonetheless found hegemonic interpretations of the (relatively conservative) programme by some who might be presumed to oppose it (e.g. left-wing labour groups), and 'negotiated' readings by others. In other words, while media producers set limits on the range of possible interpretations of their programming, in the end their audiences did not need to agree with every idea they put forward (c.f. Turner, 2003).

Although Morley's focus on television was not uncommon at this time (e.g. also see Ang, 1985; Katz & Liebes, 1986), soon enough other scholars would point out that TV's influence extended beyond simply conveying visual and auditory messages. Silverstone (1994) suggested that media were 'doubly articulated', meaning that, on the one hand, media like television indeed foreground particular ideas, but that, on the other, they have a *physical* presence that affects audience experiences as well. The TV does not just legitimise cultural knowledge; it shapes things like where and when families convene in the household (Lull, 1990). This idea was in large part what motivated researchers to take an ethnographic approach to studying media audiences as the 1980s moved forward, meaning an approach that involved spending time in 'natural' media consumption settings and employing methods like participant observation therein. Gray (1992), for example, spent time in family households to explore the use and control of the VCR cassette player. In this ethnographic approach, she found that women were less likely to exert control over the VCR, for the unequal distribution of household labour left them less time for leisure participation.

As time passed, this desire to study media consumers as they went about their daily activities only grew. There were (at least) two central reasons for this. First, media was branching out to occupy more and more aspects of people's daily experiences. Not only do people now engage with technologies ranging from newspapers to high definition televisions to interactive Smartphone apps, but they do so in untraditional settings: Someone might well watch Olympic hockey or today's equivalent of *Nationwide* on the bus ride home. Second, and partly because of this first trend, scholars began to question whether pre-formed media audiences even exist in the first place. It is difficult to identify *the* audience for the programme *Hockey Night in Canada (HNIC)*, for instance, when some might watch the live broadcast of this show, others might follow an HNIC blog, and still others might consume it through clips on a site like YouTube. Media audiences are now fractured entities, and perhaps always were so to begin with (see Hartley, 2006).

The proliferation of media, and the growing skepticism among scholars that clearly defined audiences exist, has influenced further changes in how media reception is studied. Media researchers are increasingly interested in examining the role of media within people's wider experiences, looking beyond media reception and even beyond the precise contexts in which media messages are encountered. As Alasuutari (1999) writes, the latest 'generation' of reception studies maintains an interest in programmes and programming, 'but not as texts studied in isolation from their usage in everyday life' (p. 7; c.f. Millington & Wilson, 2010a). Rather, media texts are seen as components of people's lives that influence and are influenced by what people see and do elsewhere. As we shall see, in our own research, we took interest in media consumption and its relationship to another key part of physical culture: school PE class.

The questions that remain here involve how and the extent to which SPC scholars have engaged with this tradition of reception studies. We have previously argued that there is still a shortage of studies on SPC media audiences (Millington & Wilson, 2010a); however, this is not to discount the small number of important studies that have been carried out to date (e.g. Bruce, 1998; Gantz & Wenner, 1991; Lines, 2000, 2007; Wheaton & Beal, 2003). One particular study that was helpful in designing the research project that we describe in the following section was carried out by one of the authors of this chapter, along with a colleague, in the mid-1990s (Wilson & Sparks, 1996, 1999, 2001). In this work, Wilson and Sparks were interested in how young people of different racial groups interpreted and identified with athletic apparel commercials featuring celebrity Black athletes – and what these audiences appeared to learn about race from viewing (sport-related) media. What they found in conducting focus groups with Black and non-Black groups of young males were slight, but nonetheless significant, differences in their perceptions of athletes like Michael Jordan (Wilson & Sparks, 1996), and major differences in their perceptions of portrayals of Blacks in media more generally (Wilson & Sparks, 1999).

While both groups consisted of basketball fans, and thus appreciated the sporting acumen depicted in the commercials, the appearance of Black athletes in (for example) Nike commercials resonated *culturally* with the Black youth in ways it did not among the non-Black youth. Specifically, the Black youth partaking in the study felt influenced by the style of the (Black) athletes appearing on-screen – a finding that supports the view that audience perceptions are affected in part by their (pre-existing) cultural experiences (Wilson & Sparks, 1996). More striking differences emerged in the groups' responses to questions about portrayals of race in mass media generally. Informed by their focus group interview findings, Wilson and Sparks suggested that the non-Black groups appeared to 'learn' about Blacks from media because of their limited exposure to Blacks in other parts of their lives, although the topic of 'Black athlete portrayals in media' was not a topic that members of the non-Black groups had thought much about. Conversely, the Black youth were intently aware of racial stereotyping in mass media, and expressed concern about how these portrayals might influence how other people saw youth like themselves (Wilson & Sparks, 1999).

DESIGN

Apart from their findings, what might stand out from Wilson and Sparks' research is that they relied mainly on focus groups for data collection. This left some questions unexplored, such as the following: How exactly did media inform their research participants' daily activities, if at all? And were there relationships between their participants' views on media – and, in particular, their views on racial stereotyping – and their daily activities? In our view, these lingering questions could have been addressed, at least in part, through the ethnographic approach to audience research that scholars like Alasuutari (1999) have more recently advocated for.

It was with this ethnography-influenced tradition of audience research – and the strengths and shortcomings of Wilson and Sparks' specific research project – in mind that we designed our own study into media reception. The first step in accomplishing this was to *select a specific topic or type of media*

to explore, as well as an 'audience' to partake in the study. Although in the
past researchers have often focused on a specific media text – for instance,
Morley's study on the *Nationwide* TV show – we were compelled by the
research of Messner et al. (2000) to examine viewer understandings of media
portrayals of masculinity *in general.* As discussed above, Messner and his
colleagues found that aggressive, sometimes violent, muscular and explicitly
heterosexual masculinities are normalised in SPC media, but that there is a
notable shortage of research examining exactly how these media messages
are interpreted by their intended viewers (i.e. young males). By identifying
this 'knowledge gap' in the literature, Messner et al. gave us both a 'type' of
media to examine (TV shows and films featuring depictions of physically
'empowered' masculinities) and an 'audience' around which to build our
study (teenage males). The reason we say 'audience' in quotation marks here
is to acknowledge that there is no single, clearly defined audience of the
Televised Sports Manhood Formula; we assumed we would be dealing with
young people who had differing levels of familiarity with media depictions
of masculinity.

    The second step in our research was to find a way to *contextualise our
research participants' media interpretations.* What we knew from the SPC
literature was that the masculinities promoted in media do not exist in
isolation; rather, they work *in conjunction* with other physical cultural sites,
including PE class. Indeed, researchers have found a tendency for school
PE, not unlike media, to privilege the idea that men and boys should be
strong, assertive 'winners' – something that at times leads to negative
experiences for those not living up to masculine 'ideals' (e.g. Brown &
Evans, 2004; Gorely, Holroyd, & Kirk, 2003). And yet, while scholars like
Kirk (2002) have suggested a need to consider media and PE together, we
found little research that actually accomplished this task. PE class, in other
words, became the site at which we carried out our analysis, examining how
young people's *perceptions* of masculinity in media relate to their lived
experiences of gender in PE, if at all.

    Third, *our study required a theoretical approach.* The concept of
'hegemony' is popular among scholars for understanding issues related to
both masculinity and youth experiences. Hegemony comes from the writing
of theorist and activist Antonio Gramsci. While imprisoned in Mussolini's
Italy in the 1920s and 1930s, Gramsci wrote that power inequalities were
sustained not simply by force or even economic control, but by the ability of
the dominant classes to promote cultural ideas or values that make the social
order seem perfectly natural. Those taking up Gramsci's work more recently
are not necessarily concerned with the upholding of fascist governments, as

Gramsci was, but they have been influenced by his view of the *processes* by which power operates. For masculinities scholars like Atkinson (2010) and Connell (1995; also see Connell & Messerschmidt, 2005), there is no singular, 'natural' form of masculinity, yet sites like media and PE work to normalise – that is, render *hegemonic* – the idea that particular forms of masculinity are 'obviously' preferred over others. Of course, there are opportunities to resist the social order, or partake in what can be termed 'counter-hegemony'. What scholars who study youth cultures have argued, however, is that young people's frequent attempts at (symbolic) resistance – for instance, their counter-cultural styles of dress or even their insightful media criticisms – often fail to overturn the social order as a whole (Miles, 2000; Willis, 2000). Hegemony, in other words, might concede momentary critiques of power, but substantial social change is more difficult to achieve.

Fourth and finally, to carry out our study, we needed to *select specific methods with which to collect data*. In the end, we settled on a three-phase approach. The *first phase* of the study involved focus groups with PE students on their perceptions of masculinities in popular media. In total, we spoke with 36 male students (ages 14–15), dividing them into focus groups of three to five. Each of the focus groups began with a short video viewing session, where we showed brief clips of masculinities – and, in particular, 'hegemonic masculinity' as described in Messner et al.'s (2000) research – in media. This usage of video clips is something Wilson and Sparks (1996, 1999) did as well. While we knew that not everyone in our 'audience' would have the same level of familiarity with (for instance) a clip of Mixed Martial Arts fighting, we saw this technique as helpful nonetheless in stimulating discussion. From there, the focus groups started with general questions about the video ('What are your thoughts on the video?'; 'Were there depictions of masculinity you liked/did not like?'), followed by questions about the students' regular media viewing habits ('Do media provide realistic depictions of masculinity?'). In this first phase of the study, we also asked students to fill out a brief questionnaire featuring similar questions in case they wanted to convey any views about media independently of their classmates.

In the *second phase* of the study, we turned to the students' experiences in school PE. Specifically, we spent roughly three months engaged in participant observation in the students' PE classes, with the goal of better understanding the role of gender in affecting both the organisation of PE and students' experiences therein. While focus group conversations can be recorded simply through an audio recording device, participant observation required meticulous note taking during and after PE classes. In phase two of the study, we also performed one-on-one interviews with three teachers at the participating school. Their familiarity with the students involved in the research lent further insight into the (gendered) nature of PE class.

Finally, in the *third phase* of the study, we reassembled students into their focus groups, in this case so as to pose questions about their perspectives on PE. Having this additional round of focus groups at the end of the study also provided an opportunity to discuss events or incidents that arose during our participant observation of PE classes. It also made it possible to revisit the students' views on media masculinities if needed – for instance, by asking their views on the relationship between gender, PE and popular media.

FINDINGS AND REFLECTIONS

In this multi-phase, multi-method approach, then, we were striving to go a step beyond Wilson and Sparks' (1996, 1999) earlier research on youth perceptions of athletic apparel commercials, namely by considering how interpretations of media relate to other components of young people's lives. What this approach enabled us to do (as we discuss in detail below) is identify some notable tendencies in our research participants' perceptions and experiences of masculinity. Specifically, as we moved to the data analysis phase of our study – which took place after we transcribed our field notes and interview/focus group recordings – two central findings emerged.

The first of these arose in our initial focus groups on media, in which we found a tendency for our research participants to express *critical* views on masculinity in popular films, TV shows and sports media. The portrayals of hegemonic masculinity in our video montage were met with a great deal of skepticism by virtually all of the students we spoke with, as our research participants considered hulking, imposing celebrity male figures to be purveyors of unrealistic or undesirable masculine ideals. From there, many students expressed similar disregard for the masculinities they encounter in their regular media consumption – for instance when watching TV. In this sense, the young people in our study were not only familiar with the media masculinities described in Messner et al.'s (2000) textual analysis, they were also disapproving of them in many ways.

Consider, as an example of this first finding, the views of the students Allan and Cal on gender portrayals in popular culture:

• Researcher: Does the media, you find, give you guys real portrayals of men and masculinity?

- Allan: Not often.

- R: No? How so Allan?

- A: Well, you see 'Roid Droids like the Strongman pulling trucks ....

- Cal: Or like Bowflex ads.

- A: You need the chiseled abs. Yeah, it's good to be healthy and workout and stuff like that, but I think that [they're not] healthy, [they're strong] ... [It's] excess in the portrayal of masculinity.

- R: What do you mean by excess?

- A: Like you need 500 girlfriends and all these steroids ... and a huge mansion and stuff like that to be a man. (FG Session 1; as cited in Millington & Wilson, 2010b, p. 1676–1677; also see Millington & Wilson, 2010c)

In this case, Allan draws a key distinction between muscularity and health, which otherwise tend to be conflated in popular media (e.g. see Dworkin & Wachs, 2009). While he implicitly appreciates the importance of the latter, he clearly rebuffs the value of the former (e.g. through the term 'Roid Droids', a pejorative reference to steroid use), while also highlighting the impossible standards related to sexuality ('500 girlfriends') and wealth ('a huge mansion') that accompany media masculinities. This was not unlike Gavin and Chad's rejection of the strong, 'manly man ... Arnold Schwarzenegger type of guy' (Millington & Wilson, 2010b, p. 1677), or Zach's critique that male viewers are 'trained' to be strong and unemotional. Some students even offered piercing criticisms of media 'encoding' processes, suggesting that media producers create unrealistic representations either for the sake of profit or to fulfil their own desires.

This first finding should not be taken to mean that the student participants in our research universally decried media depictions of hegemonic masculinity. There was some ambivalence in their views – for instance, when one student suggested that male figure skaters do not live up to masculine standards. Nonetheless, in coding our interview transcripts – a process by which one closely reads through transcripts several times with the goal of highlighting common themes – we found our participants to be much more eager and earnest in their dismissal of domineering male figures. This, we feel, is an important finding: Even though some media scholars have urged for recognition of young people's critical media literacy skills (e.g. Miles, 2000), the assumption that youth are vulnerable and impressionable in their relationships with media still arises quite frequently (see Giroux, 2000; Wilson, 2006).

Had our research concluded at this point, as audience studies sometimes do, we would have left our research site with a particular understanding of our study participants and their views on masculinity. As noted, however, following our initial focus groups, we stayed at our site to consider media perceptions vis-à-vis the students' lived experiences in PE, employing participant observation and teacher interviews (phase 2) and a second round of focus groups (phase 3) to accomplish this. Our second central finding arose at this time and provided an interesting contrast with the first.

Namely, there was a tendency in our second focus groups for students to *valorise* competitive, aggressive masculinities in PE – which is to say they now *supported* the masculine ideals they had previously *critiqued*. This finding was corroborated by our observations of PE, through which we at times witnessed the formation of gender hierarchies, and by the PE instructor who informed us that 'to be an athletic male is still to be pretty much top of the heap in high school' (Millington & Wilson, 2010b, p. 1680).

As an example of this second finding, consider the student Chad's relationship with his classmate Tim:

- Chad: Remember that dodgeball game we had [a few times ago] where I was telling you how I killed Tim ... I cracked him in the stomach?

- Researcher: Yeah.

- C: I was so happy.

- R: Why was that so exciting to you?

- C: Because he always annoys me ... . He's just a sack of shit! He doesn't do anything. (FG Session 2; as cited in Millington & Wilson, 2010b, p. 1679)

Chad's comments here are reflective of the fact that in the context of PE, the most imposing students could physically antagonise others if they so desired. Games like dodgeball and 'murderball', whose very purpose is to target others with projectile objects, evidently provided the ideal opportunity for students to 'crack' one another in the stomach. At a deeper level, though, Chad's comments signal that it was not just his physical strength that enabled such behaviour but also the *sanctioning* of this type of aggression to begin with. Indeed, other students expressed similar disdain for supposedly passive students in PE, for example when Clayton asserted that '[Girls are] wimps. They're afraid of the ball', and when Austin claimed that '[Girls] just don't do anything' (Millington & Wilson, 2010b, p. 1679). Once again, it is important to clarify that this finding does not capture the entirety of the students' experiences in PE, and that in our observations we witnessed instances of cooperative, non-violent play. Nonetheless, the tendency for our research participants to celebrate hegemonic masculinity is an important finding as well – one that is supported by other research carried out in PE settings, as noted above.

By taking an approach to media analysis that looks beyond 'decoding', we were able to develop a greater appreciation of the complexities surrounding young people's experiences in our contemporary media culture (Alasuutari, 1999). Without the second and third phases of our research, we might have only concluded that young males are highly discerning, even progressive, in their understanding of gender, for the youth in our research were willing to spurn the media's narrow definitions of masculinity. But by considering media interpretations within the broader context of our participants' lives, we unearthed some notable contradictions between their *perceptions* of masculinity and their lived gender *experiences*. Students like Chad and Allan were able to admonish the 'Arnold Schwarzenegger type of guy' in one context (media reception) and then valorise that same masculine archetype in another (PE). The students' celebration of hegemonic masculinity in PE, of course, does not nullify their profound media criticisms, but it does give us a sense of how seemingly powerful viewpoints can also be limited by other components of young people's lives.

Indeed, it is at this point that our previously mentioned theoretical framework becomes particularly relevant. Since it is true that the students in our research had unfavourable views of media masculinities, and since it is true that other scholars have stressed audiences' critical media literacy skills, one might wonder why our participants did not seem to 'follow through' with their media criticisms. As described above, the concept of hegemony suggests that power hierarchies are sustained when socially constructed meanings are made to seem natural and thus unassailable. This does not deny, however, that there can be criticisms of existing power structures (or 'counter-hegemony'); rather, it means that the social order (or in this case, the gender order) is so engrained that local acts of criticism often fail to overturn it. Our study suggests that because hegemonic masculinity is privileged, even rewarded, *across* SPC contexts, it would be highly risky for young people to carry criticisms of media (made in the abstract) into their real, daily lives. Gavin, the aforementioned participant in our study, expressed this power of hegemony quite eloquently: 'You have to look at what everyone expects you to be. So you can disagree with something but you'll always want to be a part of society so you have to ... go along with it' (FG Session 1; Millington & Wilson, 2010b, p. 1679). Here we see the value of employing a theoretical framework in media analyses: it allows *explanation* of one's research findings, and not simply a description of them.

CONCLUSION

Our goal in using multiple research tools was to put us in a position to consider how the various findings that emerged from our study of masculinity, identity and media *would inform one another*. The information gathered during our participant observation, teacher interviews and second set of focus groups (on PE) helped us make sense of the data that emerged in our initial focus groups (on media), and vice versa. In fact, the information from different phases of our study actually affected the research *as it unfolded*. For example, as noted above, in our second focus groups, we were able to discuss specific incidents that emerged during our observation of PE (e.g. Chad's relationship with Tim), and ask questions that referred back to our earlier focus groups on media.

But even in this multi-method approach, we did not assume that our findings represented a complete picture of the participants in our research, nor the social context we were studying. 'Epistemology' is the term given to one's beliefs about how and the extent to which the world can be known (Silk, Andrews, & Mason, 2005). Traditionally, researchers have sought to know the social world by 'triangulating' their findings, which is to say employing a variety of data collection methods so as to pinpoint indisputable truths about study topics. More recently, though, other researchers have called this idea into question, arguing that researchers themselves are always swayed by biases (much like media producers and audiences!), and that the 'truths' they uncover are thus always partial in nature (Richardson, 2003). We agree with the latter point of view, which is to say we *do not* feel that audience research provides knowledge of how media texts are understood with absolute certainty. Rather, it reveals *some* of the likely ways that media consumers interpret what they see and hear, and provides *partial* insights into audience members' lived experiences.

Recognising this partiality, audience research nonetheless retains many noteworthy strengths. In our research, for example, we contributed to a glaring 'gap' in the SPC literature whereby audiences and their diverse interpretive strategies have mostly escaped scholarly attention. As we have previously stated (Millington & Wilson, 2010a), we feel the study of SPC is incomplete so long as audience perspectives are unaccounted for, since without investigating audience views and experiences, researchers are left simply to assume how media texts are interpreted.

Furthermore, we assert that our method of analysis led to findings that are relevant outside of research communities. For example, while other scholars have suggested a need for critical media literacy programmes in PE (e.g. Lines, 2007), our finding that young people are often eager to criticise media suggests that such initiatives indeed have great potential. Based on the second and third phases of our study, we would add that critical media pedagogies should not simply strive to cultivate young people's media reading strategies, but to encourage reflection on how critical 'decodings' of media can transfer to students' everyday experiences. Furthermore, our findings might be pertinent to applied work on the role of young male bystanders in contexts where higher status males are bullying lower status ones, since some of those witnessing such confrontations might understand the root causes of such confrontations (e.g. how masculine hierarchies and violent masculinities are reinforced in sport media and elsewhere) but not have the practical tools to intervene (Katz, 2005). As these examples demonstrate, audience studies can be useful in fomenting interventions into the contexts in which they take place – something SPC researchers often regard as highly important (e.g. Howell, Andrews, & Jackson, 2002).

But there are, of course, challenges that come with this integrated approach to media analysis as well. The demands on time and resources in audience research are generally much greater than in textual analyses, though are comparable with sport production studies. Our research, for example, involved a lengthy (though certainly necessary) ethical approval process, as we required authorisation from our employing institution (The University of British Columbia), the local school board, the host school and PE instructors, as well as consent from students and their parents too. Moreover, by employing methods like participant observation in audience research, scholars must be attentive to the insider/outsider dynamics that come with ethnographic studies in general. In our project, there was a need to appear and act professionally when 'in the field' in the interest of maintaining relationships with PE teachers, and a parallel need to avoid being perceived as an authority figure by participating students, since this might compromise their candidness in focus groups. Such challenges must be met with reflexivity from the researcher(s), which for us meant attending not only to the ways that we became a part of the research environment we were studying but also how our own preconceptions and biases influenced the sorts of field note observations we recorded and our ongoing interpretations of the data.

There is also the question of precisely which lived contexts should be studied in conjunction with media reception in research that takes an approach similar to our own. We decided to study media and PE together, given that earlier research had suggested a link in their promotion of hegemonic masculinity. Other audience researchers might well take interest in different ethnographic sites, however, depending on the type of media under study and the research questions they are seeking to answer.

Looking ahead, a challenge for SPC researchers interested in media will be theorising and remaining cognisant of the increasingly blurry line between media production, texts and consumption. Indeed, 'audience' experiences increasingly involve production and consumption together, as (newer) media like video games encourage users to interpret and create content (e.g. see Hutchins, 2008; Millington, 2009). With this in mind, and as SPC researchers driven by an interest in context and cultural change, we see the need for studies that explore this relatively newfound tendency in media culture. We are referring here also to the production and consumption of content through (for example) Smartphone apps, to the increasingly interactive nature of news media (where reader responses become 'part of the news' itself in many online news formats), and to the important role that blogging and alternative forms of highly accessible media have come to play in the broader cultural landscape. While this raises important question about whether 'new methods' are needed for 'new media', what we can say for sure is that exploring the various experiences of media 'audiences' remains as important as ever at a moment when media and everyday life have become linked in unprecedented ways.

FIVE KEY READINGS

1. Kirk, D. (2002). The social construction of the body in physical education and sport. In A. Laker (Ed.), *The sociology of sport and physical education: An introductory reader* (pp. 79–91). New York: Routledge.
Kirk's chapter develops an argument for bridging research on media with research on physical education. This chapter signifies an important beginning for sociologists of sport interested in better understanding relationships between these influential sites of physical culture.

2. Lines, G. (2007). The impact of media sport events on the active participation of young people and some implications for PE pedagogy. *Sport, Education and Society, 12*(4), 349–366.
For this study of youth media audiences, daily diaries and interviews were used to assess relationships between 'interpretations of mass mediated sport'

and 'physical activity levels'. Since audience researchers working in a cultural studies tradition are generally quite open to the use of various strategies for studying audiences, this is an important study for broadening our thinking about how audience research could be conducted.

3. Nightingale, V. (Ed.) (2011). *The handbook of media audiences*. Malden, MA: Wiley-Blackwell.
A set of 'state of the art' essays are included in this recently released handbook – essays that speak to the continuing relevance of the audience in an era where the distinction between producer and audience member is less obvious than ever. The essay by Nick Couldy entitled 'The Necessary Future of the Audience ... and How to Research It' is especially pertinent for those interested in a discussion of why studying audiences still makes sense in the contemporary moment.

4. Press, A., & Livingstone, S. (2006). Taking audience research into the age of new media: Old problems and new challenges. In M. White & J. Schwoch (Eds.), *The question of method in cultural studies* (pp. 175–200). London: Blackwell.
This chapter examines the history and positioning of the audience in an age of new(er) media, and reflects on the implications of recent media-related social and cultural changes for scholars interested in studying 'the audience'. The links between the audience research tradition and cultural studies outlined in the essay are especially pertinent for readers working in physical cultural studies.

5. Millington, B., & Wilson, B. (2010). Media consumption and the contexts of physical culture: Methodological reflections on a 'Third Generation' study of media audiences. *Sociology of Sport Journal*, 27(1), 20–53.
Extending some of the key issues dealt with in the current chapter, this article includes a detailed discussion of the reasons that a multi-method approach to doing audience research was helpful in our attempts to develop a nuanced understanding of media interpretations of masculinity and performances of masculinity. We point, in particular, to ways that our 'third generation' audience study contributed to an enriched understanding of the social and cultural contexts for media viewing, the illumination of extant social hierarchies and a better understanding of the contradictions of everyday lived experience.

REFERENCES

Alasuutari, P. (1999). Introduction: Three phases in reception studies. In P. Alasuutari (Ed.), *Rethinking the media audience: The new agenda* (pp. 1–21). Thousand Oaks, CA: Sage.

Ang, I. (1985). *Watching Dallas – Soap opera and melodramatic imagination*. London: Methuen.

Atkinson, M. (2010). *Deconstructing men & masculinities*. Don Mills, ON: Oxford.

Brown, D., & Evans, J. (2004). Reproducing gender? Intergenerational links and the male PE teacher as a cultural conduit in teaching physical education. *Journal of Teaching in Physical Education, 23*(1), 48–70.

Bruce, T. (1998). Audience frustration and pleasure: Women viewers confront televised women's basketball. *Journal of Sport and Social Issues, 22*(4), 373–397.

Clarke, C., & Clarke, J. (1982). Highlights and action replays: Ideology, sport and the media. In J. Hargreaves (Ed.), *Sport, culture and ideology* (pp. 62–87). London: Routledge.

Connell, R. (1995). *Masculinities*. Cambridge: Polity.

Connell, R., & Messerschmidt, J. (2005). Hegemonic masculinity: Rethinking the concept. *Gender and Society, 19*(6), 829–859.

Darnell, S. C., & Sparks, R. (2005). Inside the promotional vortex: Canadian media construction of Sydney Olympic triathlete Simon Whitfield. *International Review for the Sociology of Sport, 40*(3), 357–376.

Dworkin, S. L., & Wachs, F. L. (2009). *Body panic: Gender, health, and the selling of fitness*. New York: New York University Press.

Forman, M. (1999). *Man on the moon [Motion picture]*. United States: Universal Pictures.

Gantz, W., & Wenner, L. A. (1991). Men, women, and sports: Audience experiences and effects. *Journal of Broadcasting & Electronic Media, 35*(2), 233–244.

Giroux, H. (2000). *Stealing innocence: Youth, corporate power, and the politics of culture*. New York: St. Martin's Press.

Gorely, T., Holroyd, R., & Kirk, D. (2003). Muscularity, the habitus and the social construction of gender: Towards a gender-relevant physical education. *British Journal of Sociology of Education, 24*(4), 429–448.

Gray, A. (1992). *Video playtime: The gendering of a leisure technology*. New York: Routledge.

Hall, S. (1980). Encoding/decoding. In S. Hall, D. Hobson, A. Lowe & P. Willis (Eds.), *Culture, media, language: Working papers in cultural studies, 1972–79* (pp. 273–314). Hillsdale, NJ: Erlbaum Associates.

Hartley, J. (2006). 'Read thy self': Text, audience, and method in cultural studies. In M. White & J. Schwoch (Eds.), *Questions of method in cultural studies* (pp. 71–104). Malden, MA: Blackwell.

Howell, J. W., Andrews, D. L., & Jackson, S. J. (2002). Cultural studies and sport studies: An interventionist practice. In J. Maguire & K. Young (Eds.), *Theory, sport & society* (pp. 151–177). New York: JAI Press.

Hutchins, B. (2008). Signs of meta-change in second modernity: The growth of e-sport and the World Cyber Games. *New Media & Society, 10*(6), 851–869.

Katz, J. (2005). Reconstructing masculinity in the locker room: The mentors in violence prevention project. In P. Leistyna (Ed.), *Cultural studies: From theory to action* (pp. 397–407). Malden, MA: Blackwell.

Katz, E., & Liebes, T. (1986). Mutual aid in the decoding of Dallas – Preliminary notes from a cross-cultural study. In P. Drummond & R. Patterson (Eds.), *Television in transition: Papers from the First International Television Studies Conference* (pp. 187–198). London: BFI.

Kirk, D. (2002). The social construction of the body in physical education and sport. In A. Laker (Ed.), *The sociology of sport and physical education: An introductory reader* (pp. 79–91). New York: Routledge.

Lines, G. (2000). Media sport audiences – young people and the Summer of Sport '96: Revisiting frameworks for analysis. *Media Culture & Society, 22*(5), 669–680.

Lines, G. (2007). The impact of media sport events on the active participation of young people and some implications for PE pedagogy. *Sport, Education and Society, 12*(4), 349–366.

Lull, J. (1990). *Inside family viewing. Ethnographic research on television's audiences.* New York: Routledge.

MacNeill, M. (1996). Networks: Producing Olympic hockey for a national television audience. *Sociology of Sport Journal, 13*(2), 103–124.

Markula, P., & Silk, M. (2011). *Qualitative research for physical culture.* New York, NY: Palgrave Macmillan.

Messner, M. A., Dunbar, M., & Hunt, D. (2000). The Televised Sports Manhood Formula. *Journal of Sport and Social Issues, 24*(4), 380–394.

Miles, S. (2000). *Youth lifestyles in a changing world.* Buckingham, UK: Open University Press.

Millington, B. (2009). 'Wii' has never been modern: 'Active video games' and the conduct of conduct. *New Media and Society, 11*(4), 621–640.

Millington, B., & Wilson, B. (2010a). Media consumption and the contexts of physical culture: Methodological reflections on a 'Third Generation' study of media audiences. *Sociology of Sport Journal, 27*(1), 20–53.

Millington, B., & Wilson, B. (2010b). Context masculinities: Media consumption, physical education, and youth identities. *American Behavioral Scientist, 53*(11), 1669–1688.

Millington, B., & Wilson, B. (2010c). Consuming media, constructing masculinities: A study of youth audiences and physical education in 'reflexively modern' times. In M. Kehler & M. Atkinson (Eds.), *Boys' bodies* (pp. 91–112). New York: Peter Lang.

Morley, D. (1980). *The 'Nationwide' audience: Structure and decoding.* London: BFI.

Richardson, L. (2003). Writing: A method of inquiry. In N. Denzin & Y. Lincoln (Eds.), *Collecting and interpreting qualitative materials* (pp. 345–371). Thousand Oaks, CA: Sage.

Scherer, J., & Jackson, S. J. (2008). Producing Allblacks.com: Cultural intermediaries and the policing of electronic spaces of sporting consumption. *Sociology of Sport Journal, 25*(2), 187–205.

Silk, M. (1999). Local/global flows and altered production practices: Narrative constructions at the 1995 Canada Cup of soccer. *International Review for the Sociology of Sport, 34*(2), 113–123.

Silk, M. L., Andrews, D. L., & Mason, D. S. (2005). Encountering the field. Sports studies and qualitative research. In D. L. Andrews, D. S. Mason & M. L. Silk (Eds.), *Qualitative methods in sports studies* (pp. 1–20). New York: Berg.

Silverstone, R. (1994). *Television and everyday life.* London: Routledge.

Turner, G. (2003). *British cultural studies: An introduction* (3rd ed.). London: Routledge.

Wheaton, B., & Beal, B. (2003). 'Keeping it real': Subcultural media and the discourses of authenticity in alternative sport. *International Review for the Sociology of Sport, 38*(2), 155–176.

Willis, P. (2000). *The ethnographic imagination.* Cambridge: Polity.

Wilson, B. (2006). *Fight, flight or chill: Subcultures, youth, and rave into the twenty-first century.* Montreal: McGill-Queen's University Press.
Wilson, B., & Sparks, R. (2001). Michael Jordan, sneaker commercials, and Canadian youth cultures. In D. Andrews (Ed.), *Michael Jordan Inc.: Corporate sport, media culture, and late modern America* (pp. 217–255). Albany, NY: State University of New York Press.
Wilson, B., & Sparks, R. (1996). 'It's gotta be the shoes': Youth, race, and sneaker commercials. *Sociology of Sport Journal, 13*(4), 398–427.
Wilson, B., & Sparks, R. (1999). Impacts of black athlete media portrayals on Canadian youth. *Canadian Journal of Communication, 24*(4), 589–627.

CHAPTER 7

CRITICAL FEMINIST/QUEER METHODOLOGIES: DECONSTRUCTING (HETERO)NORMATIVE INSCRIPTIONS

Caroline Fusco

ABSTRACT

Purpose – *The purpose of the chapter is to introduce queer feminist cultural studies methodologies. For illustrative purposes, the chapter draws upon one specific study of locker room space undertaken by the author.*

Design/methodology/approach – *The design of the locker room study is delineated, including methods of data collection and analysis: self-reflective narratives, interviews, text and discourse analysis. Issues of contextualisation and insight into the use of queer feminist cultural studies methodologies to study normative geographies are foregrounded.*

Findings – *Findings acknowledge the systems of knowledge production that cohere around gendered and (hetero)sexed normative and non-normative bodies in locker room spaces.*

Qualitative Research on Sport and Physical Culture
Research in the Sociology of Sport, Volume 6, 151–166
Copyright © 2012 by Emerald Group Publishing Limited
All rights of reproduction in any form reserved
ISSN: 1476-2854/doi:10.1108/S1476-2854(2012)0000006010

Research implications – *There is no quintessential queer methodology, which is a drawback to researchers trying to forge their way in this area. Instead, all interrogations and interpretations start from a critique of the (hetero)normative discourses and practices of gender and sexuality that take place at the expense of non-normative experiences.*

Originality – *The chapter provides an overview of queer feminist cultural studies theories and methodologies, for those unfamiliar with this post-positivist and counter-hegemonic approach. The author suggests that queer feminist cultural studies methodologies provoke us to ask the following questions: What new thoughts does my work make possible to think? What new emotions does my work make possible to feel? What new sensations and perceptions does it open up for diverse subjectivities? Such questions take researchers in new and exciting directions.*

Keywords: Postmodernism; poststructuralism; queer feminist cultural studies; cultural geography; (hetero)normativity; gender

INTRODUCTION: THE EMERGENCE OF QUEER FEMINIST CULTURAL METHODOLOGIES

The theory I call on is queer theory, particularly Eve Sedgwick's (1997, p. 3) idea of reparative critique that calls for a 'deroutinizing methodology' that shakes out the impacted and over-determined in moving from truth-value to performative effect (Lather, 2008, p. 222).

Critical feminist and queer methodologies in sport and physical culture studies have arisen out of a long scholarship in the sociology of sport and physical culture based on feminist postmodernist and poststructuralist theories (Sykes, 1998). These theories seek to challenge and 'deroutinise' (Lather, 2008) deterministic understandings of the social world (e.g. based on gender differences, sexuality).[1] Postmodern and poststructuralist theorists have developed an 'incredulity towards meta-narratives' (Jarvie & Maguire, 1994)[2] and reject universal binary oppositions (e.g. male/female, hetero/homo, normal/abnormal, self/other) as they are viewed as discriminatory scientific classifications that serve to rationalise hegemonic, patriarchal and (hetero)normative power relations[3] (Butler, 1990, 1993; Fuss, 1991; Grosz, 1994, 1995; Namaste, 1994; Sedgwick, 1993).

Modernity coincides with 'philosophical commitments, to "truth", "rationality" and rationalisation, "progress", and with the belief that scientific analysis is the means by which the world will come to be known' (Fox, 1994, p. 7). This carries with it implications of an objective, unmediated wisdom about the world, and a desire for absolute and original truth (Fox, 1994):

> Seeking structures and systems, strategies and grand narratives, structuralism has fabricated the world, to the extent that it is the world. If only the jigsaw can be constructed from the pieces of data strewn about, structuralism argues, we can have the big picture. Once we have the big picture, we can control it, change it, we will be empowered. (Fox, 1994, p. 2)

Feminist scholar, Donna Haraway (1988), calls the social scientific obsession with objectivity and metaphysical truth the 'godtrick'. The godtrick refers to Western science's illusion of infinite vision of truth that is posited as 'real', 'stable' and 'infinitely knowable' (Haraway, 1988). In contrast, '[i]n social theory, post-structuralism concerns itself with the indeterminacy in social interactions and the efforts which are made by human agents to control or define reality' (Fox, 1994, p. 163). Moreover, feminist poststructuralist theorists suggest that all grand narratives (e.g. about gender and/or sexuality) are fabricated uncritically in an andro-centric, patriarchal and heteronormative culture (Butler, 1990, 1993; Foucault, 1978; Grosz, 1994; Probyn, 1996; Sedgwick, 1993).

Postmodernist and poststructuralist critiques opened up a space for critical feminist and queer understandings of the social world. Sykes (2006) argues that the 'post-structural critique of a stable, unified humanist identity has been influential in the cultivation of queer theory' (p. 15).[4] Feminist postmodern, poststructuralist and queer theories understand individuals and knowledge production as the effect of patriarchal and (hetero)norma-tive power.[5] Methodological frameworks are then engaged to challenge 'the normative social ordering of identities and subjectivities along the heterosexual/homosexual binary as well as the privileging of heterosexuality as "natural" and homosexuality as its deviant and abhorrent "other"' (Browne & Nash, 2010, p. 5).

While feminist poststructuralism and postmodern theoretical positions have influenced social science and cultural studies research since the 1980s and 1990s, an explicitly queer studies have only entered SPC research agendas in the last decade (Ahmed, 2006; Browne & Nash, 2010; Sykes, 2006). Although scholars who use any of these 'counter theories' (Lather, 2007), and the methods that emanate from such positions, take a diverse set of interrogations as their starting point, they do coalesce around some of the following themes: a rejection of universalist theories of gender and sexuality;

an interrogation of positivistic methodological conventions that posit essentialised notions of gender and sexuality; a challenge to rigid academic disciplinary boundaries; a questioning of the truth/knowledge claims that were advanced by modern Enlightenment meta-narratives on gender and sexuality; an exploration of structural systems that enable and constrain the production of knowledge about gendered and sexual subjectivities; and a pervasive rejection of quantitative methods.

A crucial focus for poststructuralist feminist and queer theorists who take up critical analyses of cultures of domination is that research provides a platform for the emergence of subjugated knowledges. This stance allows for the political representation of multiple interests and subjectivities *if methodologies are used deliberately to unpack these marginalised knowledges* (Ahmed, 2006; Britzman, 2000; Browne & Nash, 2010; Fine, 1997; Phelan, 1994; Weedon, 1997). Subjugated knowledges may destabilise dominant knowledge production within the academy and elsewhere, and critique the social construction of cultural classification systems and lines of stratification (e.g. sexual and gender differences, racialised differences). These critical approaches – what might be grouped together as *queer feminist cultural studies approaches* (Probyn, 1996) – 'argue against an orderly, universal, and predictable notion of signification and focus instead on slippages of meaning, "floating signifiers", dissimilarity, and the instability and unpredictability of language and cultural systems' (McDonald & Birrell, 1999, p. 290).

A *queer feminist cultural studies* research approach in sport and physical cultural studies focuses more specifically on critiquing, exposing, dismantling and undermining the following: dominant androcentric and positivistic methods of a 'traditional' sociology of sport (see Caudwell, 2006 for an overview on sport, sexualities and queer theory); 'modern culture's resourceful appropriation of the body' (Pronger, 2002, p. 293); the project of boundary maintenance and differentiation in physical culture (Pronger, 1998); the 'constructedness of sexuality', 'systemic violating' compulsory sex/gender relations and 'heteronormative hegemonic discourses' in sport (Caudwell, 2006); the effects of relations of power on marginalised and 'abjected' bodies in physical culture spaces (Eng, 2006; Fusco, 2006; Sykes, 2006) and the racialisation of heteronormativity (Abdel-Shehid, 2005; Jaimeson, 2003; McDonald, 2006). Subsequently, queer feminist cultural studies researchers take up methods that will enable such interrogations to take place, most notably qualitative methods (Gamson, 2000) including ethnographies (Browne & Nash, 2010) and phenomenology (Ahmed, 2006).

DESIGNING A METHODOLOGY TO EXPLORE (HETERO)NORMATIVE INSCRIPTION/S IN SPACE

... in my methodological approach I differentiate between feminist understanding – which asks questions texts insist upon – and queer overstanding – which asks questions texts do not pose ... . (Sykes, 2006, p. 18)

Caudwell (2006, p. 2) states that the focus on sexuality in queer studies (e.g. with a focus on other socially differentiated identities) works 'as an effective challenge to heteronormativity because of branding and celebrating the marginalised and/or excluded' and, in doing so, it 'stretches' traditional methodologies. Queer feminist cultural studies methods, ostensibly, work to deconstruct the cultural teachings of heteronormative orthodoxy.[6] A queer feminist cultural studies methodology is most usually interdisciplinary and focuses on asking qualitative questions about the social and cultural reproduction of gendered and sexual identities and representations, as well as their racial/ethic and class underpinnings. Methodological interrogations might be said to adopt a Deleuzian 'tool box' approach. As Massumi (1992, p. 8) notes:

Deleuze's own image for a concept is not as a brick but as a 'tool box'. He calls his kind of philosophy 'pragmatics' because its goal is the invention of concepts that do not add up to a system of belief or an architecture of propositions that you either enter or you don't, but instead pack a potential in the way a crowbar in a willing hand envelops an energy of prying.

In my case, my queer feminist cultural studies approach intersected with an interest in cultural geography. Studies of space and place illustrate that space is socially produced (Crang & Thrift, 2000; Gregory, 1994; Lefebvre, 1991; Nast & Pile, 1998); people's gendered, sexual and racialised subjectivities are intricately connected to space and place (Bondi, 1992; Colomina, 1992; Massey, 1994; Razack, 2000, 2002; Ruddick, 1997); architecture is imbued with hegemonic masculine and racialised ideals (Blum, 1998; Dovey, 1999; Fusco, 2005; Ingraham, 1992) and that power relations and social dividing practices operate in the spaces of SPC (Fusco, 2009; Johnson, 1998; van Ingen, 2003; Vertinsky, 2004). Combing my interests in cultural geography with a critique of gender and sexuality provoked me, for example, to take the locker room as my point of critical examination. Investigating such a space from a queer feminist cultural studies perspective meant asking qualitative, ethnographic and phenomenological questions about how such a space serves to (re)produce (hetero)normativity through discursive and material practices (e.g. policy statements, informational brochures, rules and regulations about what is normal/abnormal behaviour for locker rooms). Using a queer feminist cultural studies framework, I adhere to Richardson's (2000) postmodern method of crystallisation, which 'deconstructs the traditional idea of validity ... ' and 'provides us with a deepened, complex, thoroughly partial understanding of the topic'. She continues: '[p]aradoxically, we know more and doubt what we know. Ingeniously, we know there is always more to know' (pp. 13–14). Richardson advocates an engagement with creative analytical practice ethnography (CAP ethnography) which seems to align well with a queer feminist cultural studies methodology that acknowledges the limits of the researcher's partial perspective(s) and the knowledge s/he produces.

Adopting a queer feminist cultural studies approach provoked me then to take up an array of methods to study locker rooms. Mostly, these methods might be thought of as ethnographic and phenomenological. Ethnographic observations and field notes, interviews and textual analysis would allow me to write a 'thick description' (Geertz, 1983) and interrogate the 'relations of ruling' (Smith, 1987, 1993) in the locker room and on gathering and interpreting, what Denzin (1997) calls '... slices, glimpses, and specimens of interaction that display cultural practices' (p. 247) in order to interrogate how space, desire and the body were regulated and/or deterritorialised.[7]

Additionally, *self-reflexive narratives* (my thoughts about my process of inquiry, the methodological questions or 'narrative turns' I was engaged in before, during and after data collection and analysis, and my own personal observations), as well as *video and photography*, were phenomenological orientations that could emphasise the 'importance of lived experience, the intentionality of consciousness, the significance of nearness or what is ready-at-hand, and the role of repeated and habitual actions in shaping bodies and worlds' (Ahmed, 2006, p. 2).

These methodologies were employed in order to foreground subjugated knowledges in locker room spaces. The trick is to do this while acknowledging that all stories about the locker rooms are only ever partial perspectives. In my study, then, I focused on what Britzman (2000) suggests are the concerns of poststructuralist theories: structures, practices and bodies, and why certain practices are made intelligible and valorised while other practices are constructed as unimaginable.

DOING A QUEER FEMINIST CULTURAL STUDY OF LOCKER ROOMS

I proceed by trying to get within the machinery of what I am describing – to become part of it. Taking to heart Deleuze's warning about 'applying theory', I attempt to work

through and with certain philosophical insights as from within I move forward and out
along other surfaces. (Probyn, 1996, p. 7)

As stated above, I used multiple ethnographic and phenomenological
methods – *self-narratives, text analysis, interviews, photography and video* –
in order to write a deepened, complex and thoroughly partial account of
locker rooms. Data collection took place at a university athletic centre over
a six-month period. I collected texts and interviewed 24 participants (e.g.
architects, facility managers, building maintenance staff and care-taking
staff, users). I took over 200 photographs of the spatial and architectural
set-up of the locker rooms.[8] I was also present in the (women's) locker room
almost daily to prepare for, and clean up after, my sporting activities. After
each of these visits, I recorded my observations. Through this immersion in
the locker room, I was able to reflect constantly on the pervasiveness of
(hetero)normativity.

When all my data were collected, I stayed close to my queer feminist
cultural studies approach and used deconstructive strategies to interrogate
particular discourses in order to subvert their privileged positions. Norris
(1987) states:

> To 'deconstruct' a piece of writing is therefore to operate a kind of strategic reversal,
> seizing on precisely those unregarded details (casual metaphors, footnotes, incidental
> turns of argument) which are always, and necessarily, passed over by interpreters of a
> more orthodox persuasion. For it is here, in the margins of the text – the margins', that
> is, as defined by a powerful normative consensus – that deconstruction discovers those
> same unsettling forces at work. (p. 19)

Within institutionalised systems of gender, sexuality, desire and
normativity, my deconstructive *re*-reading of the locker room asked:
What do the discourses and practices in locker rooms call on subjectivity
and space to become? And, rather than asking what normative discourses
and practices *mean*, I was more interested in asking what do they *do*, how
do they *function*, what do they *affect* and what do they *produce* (Grosz,
1994, p. 170).

My findings demonstrated that there are two pervasive discourses and
practices that were operating in locker rooms – *Archi-Texts and Body-Texts*.
Archi-Texts were meta-institutional texts and discourses that signified how a
place such as a locker room was to be administered, maintained, used and
regulated by users. These texts inscribe and prescribe social interaction
around and in the locker room. Taking up a queer feminist cultural studies
methodology would allow one to re-read the pervasive and taken-for-
granted representations on the social landscape and reinterpret them as
hetero(normative) organisations of the locker room space. For example, the

signs at the locker room entrance (men and/or women) indicate a set of rules and regulations about whose body belongs or does not belong in which space.

> At the locker room I am confronted with only two choices, to either enter the women's or the men's locker room. These kind of signs then circumscribe an entrance that corresponds to my (explicitly, if it is so) sexed body, one that marks a refusal of entry to my opposite body (Blum, 1998). The gendering and sexing of bodies (my body) at the locker room entrance is then a spatialised event. Blum (1998) states "the anatomical, then, appears to be an effect of spatial significations whereby the selection of the door tells you what you have (or lack, as the case may be)... this is part of its structural guarantee" (pp. 264–265). Thus through the symbolic representations on the locker room door the materiality of gender and (hetero)sexuality is forcibly produced (Butler, 1997), and this is constantly repeated each and every time someone enters the appropriate locker room. (self-narrative from field notes, December 13, 2002)

I also found that the Archi-Texts and their processes of inscription, the textual practices 'that insinuate the modern logos ... into the lives of human beings' (Pronger, 2002, p. 154) further constituted a set of *Body-Texts* (i.e. the embodied everyday experiences of people who administer, staff and use the locker rooms) in the locker room. Body-Texts are intimately connected with people's everyday embodied experiences in locker rooms and I was interested in how individuals' Body-Texts complied with or transgressed the Archi-Texts. What I found, mostly, was that (hetero) normative organisation of the locker room doors enabled a policing of space that had repercussions for marginalised sexual subjectivities.

> Jorge (Interviewee): I don't tend to flame out in the locker room – I act more manly. I don't speak gay, or say, "Hey girl, how's it going, that's a fabulous shirt." I don't speak to these other people like that. I don't know why, because I do it in other environments. But being in the locker room where everyone is naked, and it being men-only space, puts some conscious constraints around that.

> Hanna (interviewee): If there was someone beside me, I would become more self-conscious about my movements, the space I was using. I would try to get smaller, less intrusive. I tower over people sometimes. I feel like Frankenstein's bride. I'm a large woman so I policed myself to be more feminine, dainty, smaller, coordinated ... now I identify as lesbian and I think my naked body would produce more anxiety than my naked straight body. I don't want to push my voracious lesbian body on others so it's not a space I am interested in disrupting.

But even spatial prescriptions are contested by those who (re)imagine and recognise locker room spaces differently. Despite the inscription and prescription of normative gender and heterosexual subjectivities, locker rooms become highly eroticised spaces for some, which disrupts the (hetero)normative space of the locker room:

> Charlie (Interviewee): There are situations that people position themselves in with the mirrors in order to be looked at ... There are mirrors everywhere, you can put on a show. A lot of looking goes on because of the mirrors. You see as much as you want to, whether you're straight or gay. Men check each other out all the time. That disrupts the locker room at that point – it becomes porn.

Finally, I created a set of texts about the locker room as an attempt to get at my own subjective experiences and the messy materiality of locker rooms, and to provoke a rethinking about how the fluidity and excessiveness of corporeality in the locker rooms might demonstrate the limits of (hetero)normativity. Using photography and video, I was able to add a texture to the locker rooms that text analysis and interviews could not enable. I took images of blood, (pubic) hair, body fluids, excrement – what I called the reminders and remainders of the messy materiality of bodies in locker rooms.

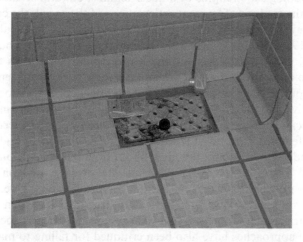

I believed that these uncanny 'objects' could queerly destabilise the (hetero)normative dividing practices of the locker room. Methodologically, it was important to find a way to represent bodily remainders and reminders because, as Shildrick (1997) suggests, 'leakiness may be the very ground for a postmodern feminist ethic' (p. 12). Leaky bodies 'captured' through everyday methods like photography present an ideological challenge to the (hetero)normative boundary and binary maintenance projects because they turn our awareness towards 'the irreducible but fluid bodily investments

which ground our provisional being in the world and our interactions
with others' (Shildrick, 1997, p. 180). Perhaps such messy reminders and
remainders of corporeality that leaks out of, drop onto, seep into and smear
spaces such as locker rooms reveal a queerness about locker rooms spaces
that can move us beyond only thinking about queer in relation to gender
and sexuality.

TOWARDS A (COMPLICIT) LEAKY METHODOLOGY

If, as queer thinking argues, subjects and subjectivities are fluid, unstable and perpetually
becoming, how can we gather 'data' from those tenuous and fleeting subjects using the
standard methods of data collection such as interviews or questionnaires? What
meanings can we draw from, and what use can we make of, such data when it is only
momentarily fixed and certain? And what does this mean for thinking of ourselves as
researchers? How does this perpetual destabilising position us as researchers and what
can we make of this destabilization. (Browne & Nash, 2010, p. 1)

The methodological strengths of a queer feminist cultural studies approach
allows for the analysis of 'current articulations of the social, the cultural, the
real as they allow or disable modalities of subjects and subjectivities'
(Probyn, 1996, p. 146); they pay attention 'what needs undoing first'
(Hutcheon, 1989, p. 23) and do not 'aim at tying all strands of life and
history into one knot' but rather attempt to locate 'the concrete embodiment
of overlapping networks of power' (Phelan, 1994, p. xvi). Problematising
the discursive and material mechanisms through which (hetero)normativity
and the social organisation of desire in the locker room proceeds, enables
the queer feminist cultural studies researcher to challenge, and hopefully
change, understandings and practices about how the acquisition of gender
and sexual subjectivities takes place at the expense of non-normative
experiences in, what Pronger (2002) calls, the production of life.

While a strength of queer feminist cultural studies has been the use of
poststructuralist methodologies that focus on deconstructing social inscriptions, these approaches have also been critiqued for failing to make explicit
how social forces, structures and discourses come to act on differently
inscribed bodies (Grosz, 1994). Moreover, although it may be worthwhile
experimenting and taking risks methodologically by 'abandoning one's
previous frameworks and terminology, of getting lost, of unsettling what
was previously secure and clear ... ' (Grosz, 1994, p. 166), casting the research
in this form means that: 'there is no such thing as 'getting it right', only
'getting it' differently contoured and nuanced' (Richardson, 2000, p. 10). A
researcher, then, has to be comfortable despite the use of multiple methods

with a sense of incompleteness, the subsequent need for continual deconstruction, and the complicity of their critique (Hutcheon, 1989). Furthermore, because queer feminist cultural studies methodologies value fragmentation, openness, multivocality (Fox, 1994, p. 7) and might be characterised by a fairly eclectic approach which 'by its very nature, impossible to delimit and define', it may be difficult to actually say what constitutes a queer feminist cultural studies methodology in the first place. In this instance, the researcher may be left with the following questions: Can I produce queer knowledge if my methodologies are not queer? Is there such a thing as queer method/methodology/research (Browne & Nash, 2010, p. 2)?

How could I write 'a [queer] vital sports text' (Bruce, 1998) of the locker room using the array of methods that I did and end up saying something meaningful about the (hetero)normative social world of sport and physical cultural studies? Using the diverse set of methodological tools I employed, I believe that my locker room study was able to, in paraphrasing from (Grosz, 1994, p. 183):

> ... start of a series of explorations of possible alternatives, possible modes of entry into and exit from knowledges that enable knowledges to be used productively in day-to-day life, in political struggles of various kinds, and in cultural creation.

A key concern for the use and application of a queer feminist cultural studies approach outlined in this chapter is the question of validity and our 'own inescapable complicity in practices of cultural production' (Lather, 1991, p. 85). Did the range of methods I used allow me to make some 'valid' statements about (hetero)normativity in the locker room? The focus in my locker room study was not about making the research and findings 'valid' in the positivist and quantitative sense but about asking: What new thoughts does my work make possible to think? What new emotions does my work make possible to feel? What new sensations and perceptions does it open for multiply situated subjectivities (Massumi, 1992)? The implication of such questions leads to what Lather (2007) has called 'a generative methodology' (Lather, 2007). In such a generative methodology, validity is a counter-practice of authority that 'disrupts any effort towards their standardization' (Lather, 2007, p. 120).[9] Such counter-practices of authority that disrupt modern science's 'own drives to orderliness and systematicity' (Grosz, 2001, p. 156) are the mainstay of the queer feminist cultural studies researcher as is remaining accountable to those bodies that are rendered abject and degenerate by the boundary maintenance body projects of modernity (Pronger, 1998) (e.g. bodies that are too fat, too old, too hairy, too disabled, too young, too black, too queer, too 'bi', too trans, too dirty and too poor).

Judith Butler (1993) suggests that what we need in a radical (SPC) demo-cracy 'is a way to assess politically how the production of cultural unintelli-gibility is mobilized to regulate the political field, i.e., who will count as a "subject", who will be required not to count' (p. 207). The methodological frameworks and tools that a queer feminist cultural studies researcher draws from may provide strategic insights into sport and physical cultural spaces in a way that opens up the 'many possible avenues of investigation and interrogation at the limits of what is thinkable' (Grosz, 1994, p. 183), and in a way that assesses the systems of cultural intelligibility all the while 'transi-tioning towards new openings in clearly contested space (Lather, 2007, p. 163).

FIVE KEY READINGS

1. Ahmed, S. (2006). *Queer phenomenology.* **Durham, NC: Duke University Press.**
This text is a major contribution to qualitative research and demonstrates how queer studies can put phenomenology to productive use. It is a particularly important text for sport and physical cultural studies researchers because of its focus on the body and space.

2. Browne, K, & Nash, C. (Eds.). (2010). *Queer methods and methodologies: Intersecting queer theories and social science research.* **Surrey, UK: Ashgate.**
A main objective of this book – a first of its kind – is to interrogate the ways in which 'queer' operates alongside social science methodologies and methods and is an essential reading for scholars who want to take up queer social science research.

3. Caudwell, J. (Ed.). (2006). *Sport, sexuality and queer theory.* **London: Routledge.**
This book brings together scholars who address gender, sexuality and queer theory in sports and physical cultures. It provides an emergent area of study and contains unique critical and political perspectives for future research.

4. Gallagher, K. (Ed.). (2008). *The methodological dilemma: Creative, critical and collaborative approaches to qualitative research.* **London: Routledge.**
A thought provoking methodology book that demonstrates how feminist qualitative researchers conceptualise methodologies and design methods to 'get at' the everyday problems being studied.

5. Lather P. (1991). *Getting smart: Feminist research and pedagogy wit/on the postmodern.* **New York: Routledge.**
This is an insightful and provocative text about how feminist postmodern researchers might turn their critical attention towards emancipatory politics. Researchers are understood to be cultural workers whose duty it is to allow subjects to speak for themselves.

NOTES

1. Hall (1997) states, 'By discourse', Foucault means 'a group of statements which provide a language for talking about – a way of representing knowledge about – a particular topic at a particular historical moment' (p. 44).

2. A metanarrative is 'an overarching discourse or position which organises other positions' (Fox, 1994, p. 162), consisting of 'stories about progress and freedom that legitimate specific knowledges and practices' (Phelan, 1994, pp. 41–42).

3. Heteronormativity describes the processes through which social institutions and social policies reinforce the belief that human beings fall into two distinct sex/gender categories: male/man and female/woman. This belief (or ideology) produces a correlative belief that those two sexes/genders exist in order to fulfill complementary roles, that is that all intimate relationships ought to exist only between males/men and females/women.

4. In the sociology of sport, postmodernism and poststructuralism are often conflated ideas. Although the conflation of these terms is often unhelpful, Weedon (1997) states that it has become a 'fact' in social theory as both fundamentally challenge modernist understandings of the world and the production and legitimation of knowledge.

5. I use 'power' here in the Foucauldian (Foucault, 1977) sense as something that is exercised in processes of social relations.

6. According to feminist and queer theorist Patti Lather (1991), the focus of deconstruction is on disruption and setting up procedures to continuously demystify modernist realities, as well as challenging the tendency for knowledge categories to congeal.

7. Massumi (1992) briefly defines deterritorialisation as 'an uprooting of the individual' (p. 51).

8. I took photographs of both the men's and women's locker rooms when the locker rooms were closed to public use and was outside of regular facility hours. Prior permission to use this research procedure was sought from the university and granted at the research site.

9. Lather (2007) suggests that ironic validity foregrounds the insufficiencies of language and produces truth as a problem; paralogical validity searches for oppositional meanings in daily practices; rhizomatic validity unsettles from within and taps into subverted knowledges and voluptuous validity moves towards disruptive, excessive and interpretations (pp. 128–129).

REFERENCES

Abdel-Shehid, G. (2005). *Who da man? Back masculinities and sporting cultures.* Toronto, ON: Canadian Scholars Press.

Ahmed, S. (2006). *Queer phenomenology.* Durham, NC: Duke University Press.

Blum, V. (1998). Ladies and gentlemen. Train rides and other Oedipal stories. In J. Nast & S. Pile (Eds.), *Places through the body* (pp. 263–279). New York: Routledge.

Bondi, L. (1992). Gender symbols and urban landscapes. *Progress in Human Geography, 16*(2), 157–170.

Britzman, D. (2000). The question of belief: Writing poststructural ethnography. In E. A. St. Pierre & W. S. Pillow (Eds.), *Working the ruins. Feminist poststructural theory and methods in education* (pp. 27–40). New York: Routledge.

Browne, K., & Nash, C. (Eds.). (2010). *Queer methods and methodologies: Intersecting queer theories and social science research.* Surrey, UK: Ashgate.

Bruce, T. (1998). Postmodernism and the possibilities for writing "vital" sports texts. In G. Rail (Ed.), *Sport and postmodern times* (pp. 3–20). Albany, NY: SUNY Press.

Butler, J. (1990). *Gender trouble: Feminism and the subversion of identity.* New York: Routledge.

Butler, J. (1993). *Bodies that matter: On the discursive limits of "sex".* New York: Routledge.

Butler, J. (1997). *The psychic life of power: Theories in subjection.* Stanford: Stanford University Press.

Caudwell, J. (Ed.). (2006). *Sport, sexualities and queer theory.* London: Routledge.

Colomina, B. (Ed.). (1992). *Sexuality & space.* New York: Princeton Architectural Press.

Crang, M., & Thrift, N. (Eds.). (2000). *Thinking space.* London: Routledge.

Denzin, N. K. (1997). *Interpretive ethnography. Ethnographic practices for the 21st century.* London: Sage.

Dovey, K. (1999). *Framing places: Mediating power in the built form.* London: Routledge.

Eng, H. (2006). Queer athletes and queering in sport. In J. Caudwell (Ed.), *Sport, sexualities and queer theory* (pp. 49–61). London: Routledge.

Fine, M. (1997). Sexuality, schooling, and adolescent female: The missing discourse of desire. In M. Gergen & S. Davis (Eds.), *Toward a new psychology of gender: A reader* (pp. 375–399). New York: Routledge.

Foucault, M. (1977). *Discipline and punish: The birth of the prison.* New York: Vintage Books.

Foucault, M. (1978). *The history of sexuality: Volume I: An introduction.* New York: Vintage Books.

Fox, N. (1994). *Postmodernism, sociology and health.* Toronto, ON: University of Toronto Press.

Fusco, C. (2005). Cultural Landscapes of purification: Sports spaces and discourses of whiteness in. *Sociology of Sport Journal, 22*(3), 283–310.

Fusco, C. (2006). Spatializing the (Im)proper subject: The geographies of abjection in sport and physical activity space. *Journal of Sport and Social Issues, 30*(1), 5–28.

Fusco, C. (2009). Subjection, surveillance, and the place(s) of performance: The discursive productions of space in Canada's national sport centre policy. *Sport History Review, 40*(1), 1–29.

Fuss, D. (1991). Inside/Out: Lesbians and gay theories. In D. Fuss (Ed.), *Inside/Out* (pp. 1–10). New York: Routledge.

Gamson, J. (2000). Sexualities, queer theory, and qualitative research. In N. Denzin & Y. Lincoln (Eds.), *Handbook of qualitative research* (pp. 347–365). Thousand Oaks, CA: Sage.

Geertz, C. (1983). *The interpretation of cultures.* New York: Basic Books.

Gregory, D. (1994). *Geographical imaginations.* Cambridge, MA: Blackwell.

Grosz, E. (1994). *Volatile bodies: Toward a corporeal feminism.* Bloomington, IN: Indiana University Press.

Grosz, E. (1995). *Space, time and perversion.* New York: Routledge.

Grosz, E. (2001). *Architecture from the outside. Essays on virtual and real space.* Cambridge, MA: The MIT Press.

Hall, S. (1997). *Representation: Cultural representation and signifying practices.* London: Sage.

Haraway, D. (1988). Situated knowledges: The science question in feminism and the privilege of partial perspectives. *Feminist Studies, 14*(3), 575–599.

Hutcheon, L. (1989). *Representing the postmodern: The politics of postmodernism.* New York: Routledge.

Ingraham, C. (1992). Initial properties: Architecture and the space of the line. In B. Colomina (Ed.), *Sexuality & space* (pp. 255–271). New York: Princeton Architectural Press.

Jaimeson, K. (2003). Latina sexualities: What's sport got to do with it? *AVANTE, 9*(3), 19–30.

Jarvie, G., & Maguire, J. (1994). *Sport and leisure in social thought.* London: Routledge.

Johnson, L. (1998). Reading the sexed bodies and spaces of gyms. In H. Nast & S. Pile (Eds.), *Places through the body* (pp. 244–262). New York: Routledge.

Lather, P. (1991). *Getting smart. Feminist research and pedagogy with/in the postmodern.* New York: Routledge.

Lather, P. (2007). *Getting lost: Feminist towards a double(d) science.* New York: SUNY Press.

Lather, P. (2008). Getting lost: Critiquing across difference as methodological practice. In K. Gallagher (Ed.), *The methodological dilemma: Creative, critical and collaborative approaches to qualitative research* (pp. 219–231). London: Routledge.

Lefebvre, H. (1991). *The production of space.* Oxford: Blackwell.

Massey, D. (1994). *Space, place and gender.* Cambridge, UK: Polity Press.

Massumi, B. (1992). *A user's guide to capitalism and schizophrenia: Deviations from Deleuze and Guattari.* Cambridge, MA: MIT Press.

McDonald, M. (2006). Beyond the pale: The whiteness of sports studies and queer scholarship. In J. Caudwell (Ed.), *Sport, sexualities and queer theory* (pp. 49–61). London: Routledge.

McDonald, M., & Birrell, S. (1999). Reading sport critically: A methodology for interrogating power. *Sociology of Sport Journal, 16,* 283–300.

Namaste, K. (1994). The politics of inside/out: Queer theory, poststructuralism, and a sociological approach to sexuality. *Sociological Theory, 12,* 220–231.

Nast, H., & Pile, S. (Eds.). (1998). *Places through the body.* New York: Routledge.

Norris, C. (1987). *Derrida.* Cambridge, MA: Harvard University Press.

Phelan, S. (1994). *Getting specific: Postmodern lesbian politics.* Minneapolis, MN: University of Minnesota Press.

Probyn, E. (1996). *Queer belongings.* New York: Routledge.

Pronger, B. (1998). Post-sport: Transgressing physical boundaries. In G. Rail (Ed.), *Sport and postmodern times* (pp. 277–298). New York: SUNY Press.

Pronger, B. (2002). *Body fascism. Salvation in the technology of physical fitness.* Toronto, ON: University of Toronto Press.

Razack, S. (2000). From the "clean snows of Petawawa": The violence of Canadian Peacekeepers in Somalia. *Cultural Anthropology, 15*(1), 127–163.

Razack, S. (2002). Gendered racial violence and spatialized justice: The murder of Pamela George. In S. Razack (Ed.), *Race, space and the law: Umpapping a white settler society* (pp. 121–156). Toronto, ON: Between the Lines Press.

Richardson, L. (2000). New writing practices in qualitative research. *Sociology of Sport Journal, 17*(1), 5–20.

Ruddick, S. (1997). Constructing difference in public space: Race, class and gender as interlocking systems. *Urban Geography, 17*, 131–151.

Sedgwick, E. (1993). *Tendencies.* Durham, NC: Duke University Press.

Sedgwick, E. (1997). Paranoid reading and reparative reading, or, You're so paranoid, you probably think this introduction is about you. In E. Sedgewick (Ed.), *Novel gazing: Queer readings in fiction* (pp. 1–40). Durham, NC: Duke University Press.

Shildrick, M. (1977). *Leaky bodies and boundaries. Feminism, postmodernism and (bio)ethics.* London: Routledge.

Smith, D. E. (1987). *The everyday world as problematic. A feminist sociology.* Toronto, ON: University of Toronto Press.

Smith, D. E. (1993). *Texts, facts, and femininity. Exploring relations of ruling.* London: Routledge.

Sykes, H. (1998). Turning the closets inside/out: Towards a queer-feminist theory in women's physical education. *Sociology of Sport Journal, 15*, 154–173.

Sykes, H. (2006). Queering theories in sports studies. In J. Caudwell (Ed.), *Sport, sexualities and queer theory* (pp. 13–32). London: Routledge.

Van Ingen, C. (2003). Geographies of gender, sexuality and race: Reframing the focus on space in sport sociology. *International Review for the Sociology of Sport, 38*(2), 201–216.

Vertinsky, P. (2004). Locating a 'sense of place': Space, place and gender in the gymnasium. In P. Vertinsky & J. Bale (Eds.), *Sites of sport: Space, place, experience* (pp. 8–24). London: Routledge.

Weedon, C. (1997). *Feminist practice and poststructuralist theory.* Oxford: Blackwell.

CHAPTER 8

EMBODIED RESEARCH METHODOLOGIES AND SEEKING THE SENSES IN SPORT AND PHYSICAL CULTURE: A FLESHING OUT OF PROBLEMS AND POSSIBILITIES

Andrew C. Sparkes and Brett Smith

ABSTRACT

Purpose – *The purpose of this chapter is to differentiate between a sociology of the body and an embodied sociology, prior to considering what this might mean in methodological terms for those wishing to conduct research into the senses and the sensorium in sport and physical culture.*

Design/methodology/approach – *The approach taken involves reviewing the work of those who have already engaged with the senses in sport and physical culture in order to highlight an important methodological challenge. This revolves around how researchers might seek to gain access to the senses of others and explore the sensorium in action. To illustrate how this challenge can be addressed, a number of studies that have utilised*

Qualitative Research on Sport and Physical Culture
Research in the Sociology of Sport, Volume 6, 167–190
Copyright © 2012 by Emerald Group Publishing Limited
All rights of reproduction in any form reserved
ISSN: 1476-2854/doi:10.1108/S1476-2854(2012)0000006011

visual technologies in combination with interviews are examined and the potential this approach has in seeking the senses is considered.

Findings – *The findings confirm the interview as a multi-sensory event and the potential of visual technologies to provide access to the range of senses involved in sport and physical culture activities.*

Research limitations/implications – *The limitations of traditional forms of inquiry and representational genres for both seeking the senses and communicating these to a range of different audiences are highlighted and alternatives are suggested.*

Originality/value – *The chapter's originality lies in its portrayal of unacknowledged potentialities for seeking the senses using standard methodologies, and how these might be developed further, in creative combination with more novel approaches, as part of a future shift towards more sensuous forms of scholarship in sport and physical culture.*

Keywords: Senses; sensorium; embodiment; interviews; visual technologies; representation

INTRODUCTION

The somatic turn in the social sciences had a number of effects. One was the development of what has been described as the *sociology of the body*. This approach made a valuable contribution by addressing various dimensions of the body/society nexus and bringing issues of the body, gender, bodily regulation and practices to the fore. This said, there were some fundamental issues that remained entirely absent from the sociology of the body that were problematic in both political and epistemological terms. For example, as Inckle (2007) points out, disabled bodies were either neglected completely or only made reference to in terms of the binaries of health and illness. She also notes that because sociologists *of* the body write *about* the body, they locate bodies and themselves within dualistic theorisations where the subject matter is separate from, and observed by, an all-knowing Cartesian subject. Therefore, as Wainwright and Turner (2006) argue, work conducted within this framework privileged and produced abstract theories about the body that ignored the fleshy, messy, material (biological) and sentient body along with the lived practical experiences of those who inhabit what Evans (2002) calls 'real' bodies.

As a reaction to the limitations inherent in a sociology *of* the body and with a view to reembodying qualitative research, calls have been made for a more *embodied* social science to be instigated that engages with all the senses. As Mason and Davies (2009) suggest:

> Social science research can benefit from a much greater awareness of the senses both in terms of its ontology (what is considered to be 'there' to research or to know about), and its epistemology (how it can be known). In ordinary and everyday ways, the senses are part of human life ... and thus it would seem at the very least peculiar to filter that reality out of our social scientific ways of knowing the world. (p. 587)

Those seeking an embodied sociology draw inspiration from work in the anthropology of the senses. Influential work here that played a key role in setting the agenda for anthropological studies of sensory experience and whose ideas continue to shape the field includes that of Classen (1993, 1997, 2005); Classen, Howes, & Synnott (1994); Howes (2003, 2005) and Stoller (1989, 1997). Together, their studies examined the history of the senses within and across cultures in terms of vision, hearing, touch, smell and taste and how these are organised in relation to, for example, the gender order. This work laid the foundation for what Howes (2006) called a 'sensory revolution' that is being led by scholars, such as, Bull and Black (2003), Paterson (2007, 2009) and Pink (2006, 2009) who are developing various forms of sensory ethnography that are influencing the contributions to an innovative new journal launched in 2006 called *Senses and Society*.

As part of this revolution calls have been made for more *sensuous* forms of scholarship in which, according to Stoller (1997), researchers lend their bodies to the world, making it radically porous, and accept its complexities, tastes, structures and smells. Building on this, Vannini, Ahluwalia-Lopez, Waskul, and Gottschalk (2010) propose that sensuous scholarship refers to research about the human senses, through the senses and for the senses. Such scholarship asks us to recognise the meaningfulness of our somatic experience of the world, 'to understand the skilful activities through which we actively make and remake the world through our senses' (p. 378).

SEEKING THE SENSES IN SPORT AND PHYSICAL CULTURE: SOME BEGINNINGS

The intellectual currents identified above have touched upon research in sport and physical culture (SPC). Calls made in the 1990s to bring the body back in to sport sociology led to the development of a heavily theorised sociology *of* the body. Here, for example, we learned much of value about the sporting and exercising body as interpreted through the analytical lenses of Foucauldian theory. This work, however, as Hockey and Allen-Collinson (2007, 2009), Humberstone (2011) and Sparkes (2005, 2009) suggested, remained overly abstract and disembodied. They expressed concerns regarding the lack of attention given to the corporeality of the body and called for a fuller engagement with the sensual and sensing body in SPC contexts. As Allen-Collinson and Hockey (2011) pointed out, while exploring and mapping cultural (and subcultural) constructions of the body and inscriptions of discourse are, of course, necessary and important research endeavours, this may result in an under-theorisation of the materiality and experiences of the lived body, both in terms of constraint and possibility. In short, to view (see) the body simply as a text is to eliminate its sensory capacities: the aural, the visual, the haptic, the olefactory, the tastes, the textures, the kinaesthetic and the visceral, to name but a few.

Attempts have, however, been made to engage with and through the senses by ethnographers operating as what Pink (2009) describes as 'sensory apprentices' in various sports and physical activities. For example, seeking to produce a sociology not only *of* the body but also *through* the body that is deployed as a tool of inquiry and a vector of knowledge as a participant observer, Wacquant (2004) takes us into the daily moral and sensual world of the ordinary boxers in Chicago. In a similar fashion, Downey (2005) takes us via his ethnography into the sensual worlds of Capoeira, where he talks of the 'apprenticeship of hearing' in training for this art and suggests that music can be a 'medium for educating the senses' (p. 101). He, like Waquant, emphasises the relationship between the body and the senses in such an apprenticeship; that is learning to sense and make meanings as others do involves us learning how to use *all* our senses (not just sight) to participate in their worlds in relation to their embodied understandings.

The points made by Downey (2005) and Wacquant (2004) are echoed in the phenomenologically informed work of Hockey (2006), Hockey and Allen-Collinson (2006, 2007) and Allen-Collinson and Hockey (2011). For example, Hockey and Allen-Collinson (2006) combine photographic and autoethnographic data to convey to the reader the particular ways of seeing, and something of the embodied feelings that two distance runners experience when they navigate their favourite training routes (see Chapter 9). Hockey (2006) extends this work beyond the visual by examining how the same two distance runners use their senses of hearing, smell and touch to learn about their training routes in different ways. Hockey and Allen-Collinson (2007) further examine the aural, visual, olefactory and haptic dimensions of sporting embodiment and note the interactive nature of the ways in which the senses operate to shape the lived experiences of the body in action. Importantly, they note how certain senses, such as smell, are mostly ignored in research about the sporting experience. However, as they point out, 'it seems plausible that different sports have different "smellscapes"; an amalgam of aromas that change according to seasonal and temporal conditions, space, place and activity. Currently, there appears to be a dearth of documentation on such "panaromas" in relation to their impact upon sportspeople and teams' (p. 122). Their attempts to challenge the ocularcentric bias in much ethnographic research in Western cultures is continued by Allen-Collinson and Hockey (2011) in relation to two distinct sporting milieux: middle/long distance running and scuba diving. Here, they focus their attention on the senses of touch, and specifically upon heat and pressure as two key structures of haptic lived experience.

Emphasising that leisure experiences involve more than the visual, Durrant and Kennedy (2007) explore its sonic dimensions by focusing on how sound is used in televised sport. They discuss a short film in which sound and image samples of televised soccer are electronically manipulated and recombined in ways that de-familiarise conventional audiovisual interactions. For them, such creative practices can destabilise dominant discourses in televised sport and open up ways for audiences to become more attuned to the capacity of sound to enrich and shape leisure activities.

In a similar fashion, Sparkes (2009) draws upon three personalised vignettes to illustrate various senses in action within different SPC contexts and explores the interactive role that the senses have in shaping his understanding and awareness of his body and the body of others over time. This project is developed by Sparkes (2010) via a multilayered autoethnographic account of his sensuous experiences as an 'older man' training in a corporate gym. Here, he explores the feelings evoked not only by the sights, smells, sounds and tastes of the gym but also by the tactile and visceral landscape the gym provides in the various social spaces enclosed within its structure which is age related.

More recently, Humberstone (2011) utilises both ethnography and autoethnography to focus attention on the embodied experiences of physical activity in the natural environment and the ways in which the senses engage with the elements. Her work seeks to show the strong awareness and connections with the environment through the senses and body, and how these feed into the emotions through physical activity in the natural environment highlighting the sentient nature of embodiment. Thus, Humberstone's embodied experience as a windsurfer are embedded in nature as she sees, smells and feels it through her skin and body as she moves in relation to the changing dynamics of the wind and sea in a given space. Likewise, in making the case for embodied and sensuously engaged leisure scholarship, Merchant (2011) examines the ways in which tourists encounter scuba diving and how they come to terms with their new surroundings as they leave behind their land-based and/or swimming techniques in the process of generating a submarine habitus. This is characterised by floatiness, minimised exertion and a consciously slow and steady respiration rate, not to mention its equipmental mediations.

Clearly, there is a growing interest in seeking the senses and developing embodied methodologies and sensual forms of scholarship within the social sciences in general and within the domain of SPC research in particular. Alongside this growing interest, and evident in the thoughts and reflections of the scholars cited so far, a number of methodological challenges have emerged that are worthy of attention if the sensorial revolution is to achieve its full potential. One major challenge, that will now be considered in detail, is how researchers might seek to gain access to the senses and the sensual experiences of others.

SEEKING THE SENSES

Seeking the senses is a difficult task. For most of the time our bodies are what Leder (1990) calls an *absent–presence* in our lives as it deals with its 'ceaseless steam of kinaesthesias, cutaneous, and visceral sensations' (p. 23). That is, we are often not aware of our bodies, they just *are*. This is particularly so in sport when rehearsed physical skills, once fully learned, pervade one's corporeality and slip beyond conscious reflection in the actual *doing*. Against this backdrop, Merchant (2011) asks, even if the body does announce itself to us in sport and physical activity, how then do we get at the sensuous, sometimes 'pre-reflective' almost 'pre-objective' detail of what happened and how people feel during the activity? How do we access fleeting embodied encounters, immanent sensations, practical skills and sensuous dispositions?

At one level, as the work of the scholars cited earlier indicates, one response has been for researchers to engage their senses in the activity under study in the spirit of classical ethnography and autoethnography. However, as Merchant (2011) points out distinct leisure, physical activity, and sporting spaces and practices are not encountered and played out homogeneously. For her, 'Each body is lived through subjectively and brings to the encounter different embodied socio-cultural "baggage" ... Just because the researcher is engaged in the activities being studied does not mean he/she is experiencing them in the same way as others' (p. 55). Therefore, if researchers, even if fully involved in the action, are not able to act as transparent communicators of participants' embodied experiences, then how might they operate as somebody who orients the participants to that which might usually remain unsaid?

In this section of the chapter, we give a *glimpse*, a *taste* or a *feel* of how some researchers, to date, are addressing this challenge. Our coverage is necessarily limited and we have chosen to focus our attention on studies that have used one of the most popular data-gathering techniques used by qualitative researchers in SPC research to gain some understanding of the experiences of others, that is the interview. Likewise, we have chosen to consider how one of the most used technologies, visual technologies, has been utilized in combination with interviews in ways that might provide routes to other senses beyond the visual. In so doing, we are conscious of the call by Pink (2009) to reconceptualise the interview as a multi-sensory event and a context of emplaced knowing that provides the opportunity to 'learn (in multiple ways) about how research participants represent and categorise their experiences, values, moralities, other people and things (and more) by attending to their treatment of the senses' (p. 81). As such, some of the cases we examine are suggestive of potential rather than actuality as the scholars, at the time, did not undertake their studies with a direct concern for the individual senses and the sensorium in action:

> The sensorium is the sum of a person's perceptions, or 'the seat of sensation' of their interpretation of an environment. The different 'ratios of sense' that make up the sensuous and perceptual means by which we come to understand and dwell in space are said to be dependent on shared cultural norms and consequently vary according to social context and geographical location (Merchant, 2011, p. 57).

In terms of potential routes to the senses in interviews, we begin by considering Stelter's (2010) notion of *experience-based, body-anchored qualitative research interviewing*. This is a specific way of conducting an interview, where the pivotal point is the participant's experiential, embodied involvement in the issues under discussion. Drawing on phenomenology and narrative studies, Stelter submits that the first-person perspective is connected to the lived, experiencing body as a way of being in the world and the construction of meaning via narrative. This said, he notes that this perspective only gives access to pre-reflective and implicit knowledge and that 'this lack of linguistic explicitness is the key challenge to making embodied first-person knowledge accessible' (p. 861). To enable researchers to assist participants verbalise this first-person knowledge and felt-sense of their bodies, Stelter suggests the following framework for the interview:

- With the help of the interviewer who adopts a non-judgmental stance and uses descriptive questioning throughout the process, the participant chooses a situation which is relevant to the research context. The researcher helps the participant 'clear the space' by, for example, asking him/her to close their eyes, breathe slowly, relax and imagine themselves in the chosen situation.
- The participant tries to get the 'felt sense' of the situation without judging, evaluating or justifying the behaviours involved. Rather, the participant should just seek a vague 'internal aura' of the situation, for example a sensation of alertness. The concern is with the present moment, the here-and-now of the situation so that the experience enacted gives rise to both *Erlebnis* (immanent lived experience) and *Erfarung* (experiential apprehension of self and situation).
- The participant then searches for a 'handle' for the concrete situation by letting a word, phrase or image emerge from the felt sense. He/she is encouraged to use language that directly refers to bodily experiences, a metaphorical and visual language that is rich in imagery.
- In their onward dialogue, the researcher and participant consider how the word, phrase or image resonates with the felt sense. They try to develop a clearer picture of the situation and the handle – a picture that most fittingly describes the felt sense. This process of resonating is repeated until the participant is satisfied that the word, phrase, image or metaphor suitably describes the felt sense.

(Adapted from Stelter, 2010, pp. 863–864).

Stelter (2010) provides an example of an experience-based, body-anchored interview with a participant who was involved in a mindfulness course and so focuses on specific bodily phenomena, such as breathing and sensations in certain parts of the body. Following the lead of Pink (2009), we suggest that this approach to interviewing can invite those involved to 'participate in multiple sensory ways of knowing by incorporating a whole range of embodied experiences and emotions into the narratives which are audio-recorded and taken away' (p. 86). As such, Stelter's experience-based, body-anchored interview as a form of social, sensorial and reflective encounter clearly has potential to explore how the senses operate and are experienced in a range of SPC settings.

According to Pink (2009), interviewer and interviewee communicate as embodied and emplaced persons, sometimes using media technologies in this process. This is particularly so with regards to the growing use of visual media to explore both visual and non-visual aspects of perception. The goal here, according to Howes (2006), is to use the visual as a means to uncover how people distinguish, value, relate and combine the senses and experience their bodies when immersed in different subcultures and contexts. A useful example here is provided by Phoenix (2010a) in her exploration of the embodied identities of mature bodybuilders via the use of auto-photography. For her, this involves 'the power of the camera being turned over to research participants to document the images they choose, and to story their meanings collaboratively with investigators' (p. 167). Having conducted an initial life history interview with twelve mature bodybuilders, Phoenix gave each a disposable camera and invited them to take twelve pictures that say 'This is me', and twelve that say 'This is not me'. These photographs then formed the basis of a follow-up interview that explored what the photographs meant to the bodybuilders via questions such as the following: What does this image represent? Why did you take this image (and not another)? Can you tell me what is significant for you here? Following this, both the interview material and the photographs were interpreted using conventional social science techniques.

While Phoenix (2010a) was not directly concerned with the senses or the sensorium in action in mature bodybuilding, it is evident from the pictures she displays that auto-photography has great potential to evoke and explore the senses. For example, Phoenix noted that her participants took numerous images associated with food and healthy eating. One of the photographs provided by a participant, named Bill, was of the vegetable display in a local supermarket. Another was of two shelves in his garage. On the top shelf are large plastic containers of bodybuilding supplements. On the shelf below is a range of malt whiskies that Bill liked to enjoy occasionally in the company of family and friends. Likewise, one participant, named Carol, shows four supermarket carrier bags filled with high quality food produce purchased from a supermarket. Another photograph by her is of a steaming saucepan on top of a gas cooker as she cooks some of the food. Such images provide an excellent opportunity to explore in interview the dynamics of taste and smell in the cultural understanding of mature bodybuilders over time, as well as their gendered and age-related dimensions in constructing the 'perfect' body for display. This is so because, as Pink (2009) emphasises, 'the photographs shown are not simply *visual* images, but also material objects with sensory qualities' (p. 93).

Likewise, while Monaghan (2001) does not refer to the sense of taste specifically in his ethnographic study of bodybuilders, drugs and risk, it is evident from the comments made by those he interviewed and observed that the sense of taste has a role to play in the construction and maintenance of the bodybuilding identity over time. That is, becoming a bodybuilder involves becoming sensitive to a range of tastes associated with the consumption of the selected foods required to fuel training sessions and build muscular mass. Thus, the neophyte might hold to the notion of food as a pleasurable experience to be enjoyed for its taste. However, for many competitive bodybuilders, due to their meticulous dietary practices, this is often not the case as their food intake is geared towards nutritional value and not taste.

Based on the data provided by Monaghan (2001), competitive body-building appears to involve learning to 'deny' the taste of food as part of a disciplinary regime revolving around dietary regulation. Yet, this denial is never complete. This is evident, for example, when bodybuilders begin the shift from 'bulking up' to dieting for 'competition shape'. In the former, to gain muscular mass, they eat copious amounts of food throughout the day and this can be 'tasty' and 'enjoyable'. However, as the diet changes in the period leading up to the day of competition, the idea is to lose as much body fat as possible to attain a 'ripped' body. During this period, the diet becomes increasingly bland and this lack of taste becomes an additional source of stress for bodybuilders during this phase of the process. Taste, then, is a sense worthy of exploration if we are to better understand the world of competitive bodybuilding. Therefore, auto-photography as used by Phoenix (2010a) and other visual media have the potential to play an important role in this exploration and could possibly have enhanced the study by Monaghan (2001) if he had chosen to use them to focus on the senses in action with his participants.

The same potentialities are evident in a special edition of *Qualitative Research in Sport, Exercise & Health* (2010, Vol. 2, No. 2) that was devoted to 'Visual methods in physical cultures'. The contributions to this volume are rightly dominated by a concern with what can be learned via visual media. However, Phoenix (2010b) points out, one reason why visual methods might be useful is that they *do* things. That is, images can evoke a particular kind of response. This evocation can bring into play and make evident the other senses in action. A good example from this special edition is the contribution by Cherrington and Watson (2010) who use video diaries as part of an ethnographic study to explore the embodied everyday context of a university basketball team.

In Cherrington and Watson's (2010) study, 15 players were provided with digital camcorders and asked to record a maximum of two recordings a day over a seven-day period. The guidance provided to them was as follows: 'Talk about your day-to-day experiences of this basketball club both on and off court. Think about who you are, how you feel, and the different aspects of identity that you bring to the team' (p. 270). Analysing the video diaries, Cherrington and Watson noted how they contained embodied, visual clues as to how participants felt about their daily lives which had the potential to open up a range of corporeal experiences to the researcher at the time of watching the diary. This then provided a rich resource for discussion in follow-up interviews. For example, reflecting on a video diary of one player that included descriptions of how first-year players were treated during their process of initiation into the team, Cherrington and Watson commented, 'we could *see* from facial gestures and the tone of his voice that the player was upset by the events that unfolded that night and we could *feel* that he was quite uncomfortable talking about it' (p. 273). Against this backdrop, it is interesting to consider what insights might have been generated if the guidelines to the players about the video diary had included an invitation to reflect on the part their different senses such as sound, smell, taste and touch played in how they felt about and came to know their bodies and identities both on and off the basketball court. Likewise, it is interesting to reflect on how each of these senses and their interactions might have been further explored in follow-up interviews using the video diaries as resource.

The potential of visual methods as a means to engage with and explore other senses such as touch and the somatic senses, including proprioception, are most evident in the work of Merchant (2011). Based on her own experiences as a novice diver watching a souvenir DVD with other novice divers of their training week, Merchant began to develop her ideas about using underwater videography to access the senses of this group. She became qualified as an underwater videographer and proceeded to film over a month-long period the tourists as learner divers as they took part in all aspects of this activity from direct skills training (e.g. mask removal and cleaning, and buoyancy control) to the free time for 'exploration' under the supervision of an instructor.

As the videographer, Merchant (2011) filmed learner divers underwater and preparing on land both individually and as a group. She then edited the film and showed it to the group with an invitation to talk freely about what they saw, remembered and felt at the time of diving and at the time of screening. The reactions of the learner divers to the film in which they can both see and hear themselves suggests that the audiovisual medium can evoke other sensory modalities and appeal to multiple senses. Video (or photo) elicitation appears to offer pathways to other senses and can bring to light, remind and encourage participants to engage and talk about a range of embodied experiences:

> By displaying the elusive character of spaces and performances, videography then can 'flesh out' reflective descriptions of events, providing the researcher and the participants with an opportunity to talk through and point out specific sensations, emotions and connections, interactively ... videography gestures toward evoking the non-representational excesses of embodied and situated experience. (Merchant, 2011, p. 60)

The point emphasised by Merchant (2011) is that if we can 'capture' and represent experience through one or two modalities, in her instance, by recording the visual and the oral, then the other senses must be accessible (to some degree) through them. Drawing on film theory, she suggests that audiences are embodied and active perceivers who do not simply watch a film, but instead, 'though memory, synaesthesia, and cross-modal knowledge generally, are capable of reconstructing and understanding what the objects and experiences of those on screen feel like' (p. 63). Importantly, it is through repeated exposure to situations, places and objects associated with sport and physical activities that people commit to memory the sensations, emotions and practices that these elicit in the body, whether people are conscious of them or not. Because this memory is located in the body, and is embodied, then, people are capable of 'knowing' things even when their engagement in them is only partial. Anybody viewing her video of novice divers, therefore, gets a partial engagement because the only senses made directly available are those of sound and vision. However, the audience members can draw on previously acquired knowledge and competencies in the act of interpreting what they see and hear. For Merchant, this is even more the case when those on screen are in fact those watching the screen, 'as the very "things" and actions represented have literally been experienced at a previous time and place by the audience members' (p. 63).

In watching the video of themselves in action, the learner divers are provided with an extension of an embodied existence by means of a re-living and differently situated view of a previous engagement with the world. Here, according to Merchant (2011), 'the meanings of the images and sounds put across to the audience are not received as signs, but rather as "expressions in the body" and so must be "fundamentally mimetic"' (p. 64). As an example, she notes the experience of one of the dive participants who, on watching the underwater footage, encountered a synchronisation of his breathing pattern to that of his former, on screen, self as it engaged with different events.

Merchant also notes how the learner divers' spatial awareness was evoked by watching themselves underwater when the perceptual horizon is lost due to the body's parallel, rather than perpendicular orientation to the seabed. These examples, she suggests, points to the potential videography offers as a gateway to sensuous scholarship, by instilling a kind of mediated mimetic response in the spectator as a previous performer of the activity.

Merchant (2011) further suggests that videography might have something to contribute to the development of a more holistic, or multi-sensual, understanding of the body performing in sport, leisure and physical culture contexts. Here, when attempting to grasp sensuous engagements with place through a video or film, the task is that of 'reading' touch, smell, and taste as well as vestibular, proprioceptive and kinaesthetic senses, by means of visual and audio material. This is possible because sensory perception is always *overlapping* and so vision and sound can be 'used' to understand how other levels of the body and the sensorium operate in and through it. In this regard, Merchant discusses the relationship between sight and touch in the form of '*haptic-visuality*' or close-vision, where the eyes themselves function like organs of touch.

The example Merchant (2011) provides from scuba diving is the sensory engagement with different forms of coral. The multiplicity and complexity of textures of coral make them particularly amenable to haptic exploration yet their sharp and abrasive contours and venoms encourages the body to maintain a certain distance. Thus, they evoke emotions. This is illustrated by the comments made by two of the participants in Merchant's study as they watched themselves on screen being preoccupied with their equipment and equalising (adjusting their ears to pressure changes) and then inadvertently selecting a bad landing place under water that was littered with urchins, slugs and rocks. One of them, named Sarah, watching herself touch a large sea slug stated: 'Eeeeeeew, that was gross! I had no idea it was there. I just lost my balance, and put my hand right on it. As I pushed off it felt squishy ... though not as squishy as it looks ... Bleuuuurrrr' (p. 67). In time with her outbursts of disgust, Sarah flapped her hands in front of her, and screwed up her face before shuddering in her chair. Sarah's comment indicates a two-fold sensuous engagement with the creatures of the sea bed. She had previously looked at slugs in enough detail to conclude that they could feel 'squishy'. Not only was Sarah reminded of this upon watching the film, but watching the images on the screen was still capable of instilling in her a sense of 'grossness' in her hands, which then rippled through her body in disgust as she shook her hands and back, seeming to rid herself of the unwanted sensation.

Merchant's (2011) study indicates that haptic-vision is but one form of cross-modal exploration provided for her participants when they watch the film of themselves. Focusing on the problems of resurfacing and 'hovering' without using their arms and legs for three minutes at 5 m below sea level in order to prevent nitrogen bubbles from forming in the body, Merchant illustrates how the *visceral* is evoked in a participant, named Hannah, as she watches herself attempt this procedure. Hannah describes her stomach flipping, getting feelings of vertigo, and her toes tingling just watching it back on the screen. Her mimetic experience of 'tingling feet' exemplify the power of memory to instil sensations or provoke acts, 'even when the "real time" and tangible instigators of these are absent, triggering reactions to registers beyond the aural and the visual' (p. 68). Clearly, for Hannah and Sarah along with the other learner divers, watching the footage of their dives evoked physical responses to the sounds and images, which allowed them to 'feel for and in' themselves the sensations instigated by an experience that had taken place in a removed location and at a previous time. The video seems to have provided a means of representing sensory experience in a way that opened more directly onto the sensorium which encouraged the learner divers to talk through their encounters as shown on the screen in rich sensuous detail.

Given the findings for Merchant's (2011) study, it is interesting to reflect on the possibilities of using other visual technologies as a route to the senses. An interesting example is provided by Houge Mackenzie and Kerr (2012) who focus on the use of head-mounted cameras as a means to generate stimulated recall with participants in post-event interviews in SPC settings. Here, video footage is obtained by light-weight, head-mounted video cameras attached to headbands or helmets where participants wear these as part of the activity. At the same time, the camera equipment also records audio sound from a microphone. The scene or the action is recorded from a point on the wearer's head or head-wear and, therefore, provides participants with a very personal view of the event they took part in. According to Houge Mackenzie and Kerr, stimulated recall using head-mounted cameras is thought to be advantageous when compared to recall from cameras placed in other locations relative to participants for the following reason. When individuals watch conventional video replays of themselves engaged in an event taken from an external perspective, they can often become self-conscious, defensive and anxious about being evaluated. In contrast, when individuals watch a replay or video footage taken from their own visual perspective via the head-mounted camera, there is less self-consciousness coupled with a high degree of immersion in the original event which allows for better recall of feelings and sensations experienced during the event.

To illustrate the potential benefits of stimulated recall using head-mounted cameras, Houge Mackenzie and Kerr (2012) focus on a study by Houge (2010) that involved a multiple-method longitudinal psychological study to explore the optimal and non-optimal experiences of participants taking an advanced river surfing course. As part of the qualitative phase of the study, five of the participants wore small, water-proofed, digital video cameras mounted on the front of their safety helmets (also see Houge MacKenzie, Hodge, & Boyer, 2011). At the end of each course section, the footage of the camera was downloaded onto a laptop computer and compiled for replay use with the five individuals. The participants were interviewed about their experiences at the end of each day on the three-day course. Here, they viewed the river footage from their head-mounted video camera and were asked to provide a real-time commentary as well as reflect upon their thoughts and feelings during the experience along with anything that influenced the experience (either positively or negatively).

As with several of the exemplars discussed above, the purpose of the study by Houge (2010) was not directly focused on exploring the sensorium at work in river surfing. Rather her main concern was with investigating flow states and motivational state reversals in this activity. This said, the comments provided by the participants in her study as they watched footage of themselves taken by themselves in the action clearly illustrate the potential this approach has for accessing the senses. For Houge Mackenzie and Kerr (2012) it was apparent that the descriptions captured the intense feelings and emotions and the sometimes rapid changes in them associated with meeting the challenge of white water adventure activities. Like Merchant (2011), Houge Mackenzie and Kerr also note that the visual and auditory cues from the video footage appeared to facilitate participants' recall of events and how they experienced them. Likewise, their comments also indicate that due to the overlapping of the senses, then, the sights and sounds of themselves in action can evoke other senses, such as the kinaesthetic. All of which confirms the potential of visual technologies to provide access to the range of senses involved in SPC activities. This potential needs to be exploited in the future.

REFLECTIONS

In this chapter, we have focused on how visual and audiovisual media might be used by qualitative researchers as a means during interviews to access senses other than vision and sound and how they are used in combination with SPC. In choosing this focus, some might feel that we are reinforcing the ocular-centric bias that has historically pervaded western cultures and academic practice in the socials sciences. This is not the case. As we have illustrated in the cases discussed above, and as Pink (2009) has argued, given the interconnectedness of the senses and the embodied, emplaced nature of viewing video or photographs, then these can be utilised as routes to a range of other senses and to multi-sensorial knowing. This is as true for the participants in a study as for the ethnographer immersing him or herself in a given subcultural setting. However, as we have indicated above, this is not an easy process to achieve and requires a raised awareness on the part of the researcher regarding the senses and sensorium as an integral part of their studies rather than as an afterthought.

Our choice to focus primarily on visual methods in this chapter is also a pragmatic one. Given that researching the senses is in its infancy in research into SPC, it seems to make sense to start with, first, a method of data gathering that researchers use frequently (i.e. the interview) and, second, a technology that is not only readily available but increasingly used by qualitative researchers (particularly ethnographers) in their work (i.e. video and photographs). As Pink (2009) comments, 'there is an increasing use of visual methods and media in ethnographic research and representation. Photographs are now widely used in publications, at least among visual sociologists and anthropologists, documentary videos are frequently made, and multimedia CD, DVD and online texts are an emergent representational form' (p. 99). That is, both researchers and participants are familiar with audiovisual media and technology which makes it more likely that their use would be acceptable in a study.

In terms of starting with what the research community is familiar with, Sparkes (2009) also adopts a pragmatic stance in assisting students on research methods courses to become more aware of the senses as both a way of knowing and a topic of inquiry in SPC. On such courses, he suggests that it might be useful to encourage students to get to know the same location over time in different ways using different senses. For example, task one might be to visit a gym and describe it in terms of what is seen via the use of photographs and field notes. Task two, on another day, might be to go in and describe the soundscape of the same gym in terms of the role that sound plays. On another occasion, the focus will be on the skinscape and how touch and textures work in the gym to create and sustain meaning. Likewise, the senses of smell (the panaroma) and taste would be the focus of attention on different days. The purpose of these tasks is to reawaken the senses in the budding ethnographic researcher and to help them realise that all the senses are involved in understanding the life of the gym or any other location. As part of this reawakening crucial questions can then be raised about how the senses interact in various combinations and hierarchies to shape the experiences and meanings of those involved in terms of various categories, such as gender, ethnicity, disability, age and sexual orientation.

Seeking the senses, as we have indicated, is no easy task. Even if this seeking is successful, another challenge emerges for the embodied sociologist who, according to Inckle (2010), engages in the 'messy, complex and contradictory factors at play in human experience, as well as the essentially emotive, corporeal and intersubjective, visceral, sentient nature of our being' (p. 35). This involves how we represent the complexities of the senses and the sensorium in action. This challenge is made evident in the following reflection by Wacquant (2004) on how he might describe to readers the sensuous intoxification of apprentice boxers and the interplay of the senses in their conversion to the world of prize fighting, in expressive forms suitable to communicating it without in the process annihilating its most distinctive properties:

> To give the proposition its full force, one would need to be able to capture and convey at once the odors (the heady smell of liniment sniffed full force, the sweat hanging in the air, the stink of the situp table, the leathery scent of the gloves); the cadenced 'thump' of punches against bags and the clanking of chains they hang from, each bag having its own sound, each drill its tonality, each boxer his own manner of accenting the machine gun-like rattle of the speed bag; the light 'tap-tap' or frantic galloping of feet on the wooden floor with the skipping rope, or the muffled squeak let out as they move gingerly on the canvas of the ring; the rhythmic puffing, hissing, sniffing, blowing, and groaning characteristic of each athlete; and especially the collective layout and synchronization of the bodies in the space of the gym, whose mere sight suffices to wield lasting pedagogical effects; not to forget the temperature, whose variation and intensity are not least relevant properties of the room. The combination of all these elements produces a sort of *sensuous intoxification* that is key to the education of the apprentice boxer. (Wacquant, 2004, pp. 70–71)

To meet this formidable challenge clearly requires something beyond the format of the *realist tale* and its standard conventions that currently dominates much qualitative writing in SPC (Sparkes, 2002). As Hockey and Allen-Collinson (2007), Humberstone (2011), Pink (2009), Sparkes (2009) and Vannini et al. (2010) argue, to convey the senses and the sensorium in action, we need to develop more evocative strategies of representation, that is to write sensuously.

Reflecting with irony on the bloodless and disembodied writing that characterises much ethnographic work on the body, Stoller (1997) recognises that the analysis of complex philosophical and political issues often requires intricate arguments expressed in densely packed discourse. But, he argues, this should not necessarily exclude sensuous expression: 'Put another way, discussions of the sensuous body require sensuous scholarship in which writers tack between the analytical and the sensible, in which embodied form as well as disembodied logic constitute scholarly argument' (p. xv). Accordingly, Stoller (1989) suggests that stylistic changes in the writing of ethnographies to include, for example, rich sensory description and vivid metaphors, have the potential to open up the world to a multi-sensory exploration. Talking of *tasteful* ethnographies he notes how they mix an assortment of ingredients, 'dialogue, description, metaphor, metonomy, synecdoche, irony, smells, sights, and sounds – to create a narrative that savors the world of the Other' (p. 32). Given that most social scientists are trained to write analytically and less so evocatively, this shift may be problematic for many, even for those with good intentions. As Vannini et al. (2010) note, scholars who wish to pass as sensuous scholars 'feel they must provide scholarly interpretation and conceptual arguments, and these rhetorical strategies inevitably displace sensuous description' (p. 380).

Importantly, Stoller (1989, 1997) does not call for the abandonment of analytical writing as a mode of representing the senses and the sensorium. Rather he suggests an interweaving of the theoretical and the experiential in sensory ethnography that utilises various registers and genres to move between the 'intelligible' and the 'sensible' and between embodied form as well as the disembodied logic that constitutes scholarly argument. Likewise, Vannini et al. (2010) maintain that sensuous scholarship is Janus-faced. On one side, it attempts to gratify the senses of the audiences. On the other side, it speaks to their 'minds' through analysis and interpretation. Rather than selecting one side over the other, or seeing the two sides as contradictory, they believe that the authentic complexity of sensuous scholarship can only be evoked through the dialectics of prose and poetry of analysis and description. Vannini et al. suggest that one possible strategy to accomplish this is via the *somatic layered account* that is proportionately prosaic and poetic:

> A somatic layered account draws upon multiple forms of consciousness or ways of knowing, such as, the embodied, the somatic, the affective, the imaginative, the linguistic and the nonsymbolic, and the intellectual and analytical. In other words, the somatic layered account speaks both to the interpretive lexicon of theory and the affective and somatic register of sensations and emotions. It touches upon both emotion and cognition. It makes use of linguistic metaphors, but it does not dismiss the role of iconic and indexical forms of signification. It is conceptual and analytical, but it also recognizes the mystifying, nonrepresentational power of enchantment. And it recognizes both the reflexive somatic work of research participants and researchers. (Vannini et al., 2010, p. 380)

In presenting their participant observation findings of performing taste at wine festivals, Vannini et al. (2010) suggest six strategies that authors can use to write somatically so that the key characteristics of *indeterminacy, non-representationality, contingency, emergence, dialectics* and *locality* might be achieved in a somatic layered account. They also consider how such accounts might be organised prior to presenting their findings through an interweaving of somatic, narrative and evocative descriptions of wine tasting coupled with an interdisciplinary and theoretically diverse analysis of this activity. Such work serves as a useful starting point for dialogue among those who seek to capture the somatic dimensions of material culture without abdicating the need to sociologise it.

Against this backdrop, it is interesting to note how some scholars in SPC have utilised some aspects of a somatic layered account in their work. For example, in his autoethnographic account of his movement from a performance to an impaired body, Sparkes (2003) combines vignettes, archive material in the form of public statements about his sporting body (that he cannot remember), flashbacks and poems to evoke aspects of his sensory experiences. Each of these are juxtaposed with his 'academic voice' that suggests analytical interpretations that the reader might consider. A more recent example is provided by Humberstone (2011) who draws on ethnography and autoethnography to explore the interrelationship of space, the elements and the embodied experiences of water-based physical activity. While the majority of her paper might be described as analytical in nature, the focal point for this is a short story and a poem about Humberstone's own windsurfing experiences that are used to evoke a sense of the interlinking of the physical and affective sensations and the mobile environment in which she is sensually immersed. Thus, once again the strategy of inviting the reader into the sensuality of the body in action and then moving back to adopt a more reflective and analytical stance has been used to good effect.

Clearly, written texts that call upon different genres of representation have a part to play in seeking the senses in SPC. However, as Pink (2009) and Sparkes (2002, 2009) point out, this does not exhaust the possibilities and writing is not the superior or exclusive medium for ethnographic representation. For example, given the immense difficulties of representing the sonic landscape in written form, Sparkes suggests the use of ethnodrama or ethno-theatre. Here, data gathered in the field is transformed into theatrical scripts and performance pieces where the sights, sounds and feelings from the field can be reconstructed in context before an audience. Likewise, given the technology now available to researchers, Pink provides a number of examples of how visual ethnographers are developing audiovisual representations that are intended to invoke the sensorial, affective and aesthetic dimensions of the lives and environments of the participants in their research.

While Pink (2009) also provides examples of those who use audio-recording to develop soundscape compositions for research purposes, she acknowledges that it remains difficult to imagine how an ethnographer might represent olfactory experiences, let alone reproduce them. Yet such experimentation is taking place in the arts. As Pink comments, 'Accompanied by a strong interest in the senses among contemporary artists, this mix of more established and emergent ethnographic genres and styles and sensory arts practice offers ethnographers a series of inspiring models' (p. 153). It would seem sensible, therefore, for researchers seeking the senses in SPC to engage with those working in the arts with a view to developing collaborative and productive relationships so that both domains can learn from each other in the future.

In closing, we wish to acknowledge that seeking the senses using embodied methodologies is in its infancy in the field of SPC. This said, as the works of the scholars focused on in this chapter have indicated, a start has been made on this venture. There is much that can be learned along the way from colleagues in other areas such as anthropology, sociology and the arts whose work can provide a valuable resource. Engaging with and through the senses in our research endeavours is no easy task and we have identified a number of challenges in terms of the adequacy of existing methods and genres of representation for communicating about the senses and the sensorium. These challenges are not, however, insurmountable and the benefits of meeting them are many – not least because the development of a more sensory research agenda along with sensual scholarship invites new forms of knowing and routes into the experiences of others and ourselves. The results, as Pink (2009) emphasises, can 'inspire new layers of knowing which, when interrogated theoretically, can challenge, contribute to and shift understandings conventional to written scholarship' (p. 153). With this in mind, we look forward to how the senses are addressed in the future by those researching in the field of SPC.

FIVE KEY READINGS

1. Sparkes, A. (2009). Ethnography and the senses: Challenges and possibilities. *Qualitative Research in Sport, Exercise & Health, 1*(1), 21–35. The author begins with three personalised vignettes to illustrate his senses in action within different sports-related contexts. Questions are then raised regarding the historical elevation of sight over the other senses in ethnography and the impact this has had on how we understand the social world with, in and through our bodies. Having provided a useful review of key literature, the case is then made for a more balanced consideration of various forms of embodiment that include the senses of sound, smell, touch and taste. How these senses are engaged in sport and physical activity settings is then focused on in detail.

2. Merchant, S. (2011). The body and the senses: Visual methods, videography and the submarine sensorium. *Body & Society*, *17*(1), 53–72.
This paper adopts a much needed interdisciplinary approach to tackle the challenge of collecting and analysing embodied, sensuous and pre-reflective 'data' by advocating the value of integrating videography into research methodologies. The author examines how underwater videography footage that features scuba divers coming to terms with their surroundings might be utilised with those involved as the divers featured in the film, and as watchers of the film to engage with, evoke and represent the 'unrepresentable' senses, such as touch and the somatic senses.

3. Allen-Collinson, J., & Hockey, J. (2011). Feeling the way: Notes towards a haptic phenomenology of distance running and scuba diving. *International Review for the Sociology of Sport*, *46*, 330–345.
Drawing on insights derived from existential phenomenology, this paper contributes to our understanding of the sensory dimensions of the lived sporting body by focusing on two distinct sporting milieux: middle/long distance running and scuba diving. The authors stress that these activities take place within particular geographical areas and social spaces that both shape and are shaped by the embodied sporting activities that take place within them. Next, as part of an ongoing challenge to the high degree of ocular-centrism in the social sciences, the authors explore the complex and multifaceted dynamics of the much-neglected sense of touch, giving particular attention to heat and pressure as two key structures of haptic lived experience.

4. Humberstone, B. (2011). Embodiment and social and environmental action in nature-based sport: Spiritual spaces. *Leisure Studies*, *30*(4), 495–512.
This paper explores the interrelationship of space, the elements and the embodied experiences of water-based physical activity. It uses alternative forms of research and representation to draw out the embodied nature of the experiences in exploring the practices of windsurfing among communities of windsurfers. The author uses both ethnography and autoethnography to

illuminate the connections between the flesh, affects, emotions and the senses as the body engages with natural elements. Her embodied experience as a windsurfer are embedded in nature as she sees, smells and feels it through her skin and body as she moves in relation to the changing dynamics of the wind and sea in a given space. Importantly, in engaging with expressions of spirituality and the speculative notion of kinetic empathy, the author is able to propose the concept of body pedagogics as analytically useful in exploring social and environmental action in local and global spaces.

5. Vannini, P., Ahluwalia-Lopez, G., Waskul, D., & Gottschalk, S. (2010). Performing taste at wine festivals: A somatic layered account of material culture. *Qualitative Inquiry*, *16*(5), 378–396.
In this paper, the authors reflect on one particular genre of sensuous scholarship that seeks to recognise the meaningfulness of our somatic experience of the world, and to understand the skilful activities through which we actively make and remake our world through our senses. The genre they focus on as defined by them is the somatic layered account. Drawing on data generated from participant observation at wine festivals at a number of sites, the authors examine how people express taste sensations and preferences to others, as well as the role wine's material properties play in these social dramas. In formulating and developing the concepts of somatic accounts, taste vocabularies and somatic joint acts, the authors contribute to a growing understanding of the social aspects of the senses and of sensations, as well as how people perceive the material world, and the sense of taste in particular, in active and reflexive ways.

REFERENCES

Allen-Collinson, J., & Hockey, J. (2011). Feeling the way: Notes towards a haptic phenomenology of distance running and scuba diving. *International Review for the Sociology of Sport*, *46*, 330–345.
Bull, M., & Black, L. (Eds.). (2003). *The auditory culture reader*. Oxford: Berg.
Cherrington, J., & Watson, B. (2010). Shooting a diary, not just a hoop: Using video diaries to explore the embodied everyday contexts of a university basketball team. *Qualitative Research in Sport, Exercise & Health*, *2*, 267–281.
Classen, C. (1993). *Worlds of sense: Exploring the senses in history and across cultures*. London: Routledge.
Classen, C. (1997). Engendering perceptions: Gender ideologies and sensory hierarchies in Western history. *Body & Society*, *3*, 1–19.
Classen, C. (Ed.). (2005). *The book of touch*. Oxford: Berg.

Classen, C., Howes, D., & Synnott, A. (1994). *Aroma: The cultural history of smell*. London: Routledge.

Downey, G. (2005). *Learning Capoeira: Lessons in cunning from an Afro-Brazilian art*. New York: Oxford University Press.

Durrant, P., & Kennedy, E. (2007). Sonic sport: Sound art in leisure research. *Leisure Sciences*, *29*, 181–194.

Evans, M. (2002). Real bodies: An introduction. In M. Evans & E. Lee (Eds.), *Real bodies: A sociological introduction* (pp. 1–15). London: Palgrave.

Hockey, J. (2006). Sensing the run: The senses and distance running. *Senses and Society*, *1*, 183–202.

Hockey, J., & Allen-Collinson, J. (2006). Seeing the way: Visual sociology and the distance runner's perspective. *Visual Studies*, *21*, 70–81.

Hockey, J., & Allen-Collinson, J. (2007). Grasping the phenomenology of sporting bodies. *International Review for the Sociology of Sport*, *42*, 115–131.

Hockey, J., & Allen-Collinson, J. (2009). The sensorium at work: The sensory phenomenology of the working body. *The Sociological Review*, *57*, 217–239.

Houge Mackenzie, S., & Kerr, J. (2012). Head-mounted cameras and stimulated recall in qualitative sport research. *Qualitative Research in Sport, Exercise and Health*, *4*, 51–61.

Howes, D. (2003). *Sensual relations*. Ann Arbor, MI: University of Michigan Press.

Howes, D. (Ed.). (2005). *Empire of the senses*. London: Berg.

Howes, D. (2006). Charting the sensorial revolution. *Senses & Society*, *1*, 113–118.

Houge, S. (2010). *Reversal theory and flow: Toward an integrated framework of optimal experiences in adventure activities*. Unpublished PhD thesis. University of Otago, Dunedin, New Zealand.

Houge MacKenzie, S., Hodge, K., & Boyer, M. (2011). Expanding the flow model in adventure activities: A reversal theory perspective. *Journal of Leisure Research*, *4*, 519–544.

Humberstone, B. (2011). Embodiment and social and environmental action in nature-based sport: Spiritual spaces. *Leisure Studies*, *30*, 495–512.

Inckle, K. (2007). *Writing on the body? Thinking through gendered embodiment and marked flesh*. Newcastle Upon Tyne: Cambridge Scholars Publishing.

Inckle, K. (2010). Telling tales? Using ethnographic fictions to speak embodied truth. *Qualitative Research*, *10*, 27–47.

Leder, D. (1990). *The absent body*. Chicago, IL: University of Chicago Press.

Mason, J., & Davies, K. (2009). Coming to our senses: A critical approach to sensory methodology. *Qualitative Research*, *9*, 587–603.

Merchant, S. (2011). The body and the senses: Visual methods, videography and the submarine sensorium. *Body & Society*, *17*, 53–72.

Monaghan, L. (2001). *Bodybuilding, drugs and risk*. London: Routledge.

Paterson, M. (2007). *The sense of touch: Haptics, affect and technology*. Oxford: Berg.

Paterson, M. (2009). Haptic geographies: Ethnography, haptic knowledges and sensuous dispositions. *Progress in Human Geography*, *33*, 766–788.

Phoenix, C. (2010a). Auto-photography in aging studies: Exploring issues of identity construction in mature bodybuilders. *Journal of Aging Studies*, *24*, 167–180.

Phoenix, C. (2010b). Seeing the world of physical culture: The potential of visual methods for qualitative research in sport and exercise. *Qualitative Research in Sport, Exercise & Health*, *2*, 93–108.

Pink, S. (2006). *The future of visual anthropology: Engaging the senses.* Oxford: Taylor & Francis.

Pink, S. (2009). *Doing sensory ethnography.* London: Sage.

Sparkes, A. (2002). *Telling tales in sport & physical activity: A qualitative journey.* Champaign, IL: Human Kinetics Press.

Sparkes, A. (2003). From performance to impairment: A patchwork of embodied memories. In J. Evans, B. Davies & J. Wright (Eds.), *Body knowledge and control* (pp. 157–172). London: Routledge.

Sparkes, A. (2009). Ethnography and the senses: Challenges and possibilities. *Qualitative Research in Sport, Exercise & Health, 1,* 21–35.

Sparkes, A. (2010). Performing the ageing body and the importance of place: Some brief autoethnographic moments. In B. Humberstone (Ed.), *'When I am Old ...' third age and leisure research: Principles and practice* (Vol. 108, pp. 21–32). Eastbourne, UK: LSA publication, Leisure Studies Association.

Stelter, R. (2010). Experience-based, body-anchored qualitative research interviewing. *Qualitative Health Research, 20,* 859–867.

Stoller, P. (1989). *The taste of ethnographic things.* Philadelphia, PA: University of Pennsylvania Press.

Stoller, P. (1997). *Sensuous scholarship.* Philadelphia, PA: University of Pennsylvania Press.

Vannini, P., Ahluwalia-Lopez, G., Waskul, D., & Gottschalk, S. (2010). Performing taste at wine festivals: A somatic layered account of material culture. *Qualitative Inquiry, 16,* 378–396.

Wacquant, L. (2004). *Body and soul: Notebooks of an apprentice boxer.* Oxford: Oxford University Press.

Wainwright, S., & Turner, B. (2006). 'Just crumbling to bits'? An exploration of the body, ageing, injury and career in classical ballet dancers. *Sociology, 40,* 237–255.

CHAPTER 9

AUTOETHNOGRAPHY: SITUATING PERSONAL SPORTING NARRATIVES IN SOCIO-CULTURAL CONTEXTS

Jacquelyn Allen-Collinson

ABSTRACT

Purpose – *To introduce autoethnography as an innovative research approach within sport and physical culture, and consider its key tenets, strengths and weaknesses. For illustrative purposes, the chapter draws upon two specific autoethnographic research projects on distance running – one collaborative and one solo.*

Design/methodology/approach – *The design of the two projects is delineated, including methods of data collection and analysis: tape-recorded field and 'head' notes, personal and analytic logs, phenomenological, thematic and narrative data analysis. Issues of representation are addressed and the chapter explores salient, but often-overlooked, ethical considerations in undertaking autoethnographic research.*

Findings – *Key findings of two research projects are presented, cohering around issues of identity construction and identity work, together with lived body and sensory experiences of distance running.*

Qualitative Research on Sport and Physical Culture
Research in the Sociology of Sport, Volume 6, 191–212
Copyright © 2012 by Emerald Group Publishing Limited
All rights of reproduction in any form reserved
ISSN: 1476-2854/doi:10.1108/S1476-2854(2012)0000006012

Research limitations/implications – *The limitations of using an autoethnographic approach are discussed, including in relation to fulfilling traditional, positivistic judgment criteria such as validity, reliability and generalisability; more appropriate criteria are proposed, particularly in relation to evocative autoethnographies. Novel forms of the genre: collaborative autoethnography and autophenomenography, are suggested as future directions for autoethnographic research in SPC.*

Originality/value – *The chapter provides a succinct introduction to the use of autoethnography in sport and physical culture, for those unfamiliar with the genre. The author also suggests an innovative variation – autophenomenography.*

Keywords: Autoethnography; collaborative autoethnography; autophenomenography; distance running; embodiment

INTRODUCTION

This chapter considers the use of autoethnography as a relatively novel research methodology within the range of qualitative forms utilised in research on sport and physical culture (SPC); a research approach that is enjoying growing popularity. After introducing autoethnography for those unfamiliar with its tenets and forms, I consider how, as researchers, we might set about designing a SPC project using autoethnography. For illustrative purposes, the chapter portrays two specific research projects, a collaborative autoethnographic study of the injury and rehabilitative process encountered by two distance runners suffering from long-term knee injuries, and an authoethnography of female distance running. Here, I shall be focusing upon the research design and execution of the projects, including methods of data collection, analysis and representation, together with some salient ethical considerations. The data and findings are also briefly considered (see Allen-Collinson & Hockey, 2001). In conclusion, I consider some of the strengths and weaknesses of the autoethnographic approach, and suggest some future developments and exciting new applications in SPC research. First then, we consider what autoethnography is and how it has challenged research orthodoxies.

WHAT IS AUTOETHNOGRAPHY?

Arising out of the 'crisis of representation' (Denzin & Lincoln, 2000) within 'realist' qualitative research more widely, autoethnography has challenged some of the very foundations and key tenets of more traditional forms of research in its requirement for the researcher explicitly to situate and 'write in' her/himself as a key player within a research account. This stands in stark contrast to more traditional notions of the researcher/author as a distanced, 'neutral', impartial and 'uninvolved' observer and recorder of the ethnographic field. Indeed, it is still considered somewhat of a contentious genre within some quarters of the more traditional social science community, due to its analytic focus upon the researcher's self rather than primarily on research 'others'. Some critics view it with deep suspicion and a high degree of scepticism, accusing autoethnographers of indulging in navel-gazing and introspection, and of generating something more akin to autobiographical writing than to scholarly, rigorous, 'scientific' research. Despite its detractors, however, autoethnography has generated enthusiastic support from researchers interested in, and committed to discovering new, innovative ways of portraying and evoking the lived experience of engaging in sport and physical culture, particularly corporeally-based experiences. For those with a background in sociological or anthropological ethnographic research in sport, for example, autoethnography represents an exciting, challenging, innovative variation of ethnography. Here, ethnographic research methods, analysis and insight are used to portray the researcher's own personal, lived experience of a culture.

In general, then, autoethnography is a research approach which draws upon the researcher's own personal lived experience, specifically in relation to the culture (and subcultures) of which s/he is a member. As Reed-Danahay (1997, p. 2) neatly encapsulates, autoethnography synthesises postmodern ethnography (where realist conventions and value neutrality are called into question) and postmodern autobiography (in which the idea of the coherent, individual self is similarly called into question); a demanding synthesis. The researcher, in her/his social interaction with others, is the subject of the research, thus blurring putative distinctions between the personal and the social, and between self and other (Ellis & Bochner, 1996; Reed-Danahay, 1997). Autoethnographers thus engage personally with the dialectics of subjectivity and (sub)culture, with different authors placing different emphases on the three key components of autoethnography: the auto, the self (*autos*); the ethno, 'race' or nation (*ethnós*) – nowadays more usually applied to a socio-cultural group; and the graphy, the writing (*graphein*) or other form of representation.

In autoethnography, the roles of researcher and participant coalesce so that the researcher's own experiences *qua* member of a social group and within social contexts are subject to analysis, in order to produce richly textured, often powerfully evocative research accounts or even performances (e.g., Spry, 20010) of lived experience. Autoethnographers thus occupy a dual, and often highly demanding, role as both member of the social world under study and researcher of that same world (Anderson, 2006). This demands of the autoethnographic researcher high levels of critical awareness and reflexivity and, many of us would add, self-discipline. Of particular interest to autoethnographers in sport and physical culture has been a focus on embodiment and lived sporting experience, together with the emotional dimension of engagement in physical cultures. Autoethnographers seek systematically, rigorously and analytically to portray their own conscious-ness and emotions, to "open up the realm of the interior and the personal" (Fiske, 1990, p. 90). This aim can, perhaps unsurprisingly, open up the autoethnographer to charges of narcissistic self-indulgence from those working from a more traditional research perspective. It can also initiate a challenging, intellectually demanding and emotionally painful voyage of self-investigation ... it is not for the faint-hearted.

A key feature of autoethnography is that the researcher's own personal experiential narrative is 'written in' (Tedlock, 1991), explicitly, in rigorous and analytic fashion as a central, fundamental and integral part of the research process, rather than as a subsidiary, confessional 'aside', which was often the case with many 'classic' ethnographies. Some autoethnographers have also engaged with novel (at least within the social sciences) repres-entational forms, such as poetry, ethnodrama, fiction and performance (Spry, 2001). For, as Richardson (1994, p. 516) highlights: "Writing is also a way of "knowing" – a method of discovery and analysis. By writing in different ways, we discover new aspects of our topic." Autoethnographic narratives thus often contrast starkly with more traditional forms of social-scientific writing, on a whole series of dimensions (see Ellis & Bochner, 2000, p. 744), including the blurring of the researcher/researched distinction, and attempts to write evocatively, to engage the reader emotionally and empathetically, and to resonate with the reader's own experiences.

The focus upon self and the degree of departure from more established realist/neo-realist ethnographic conventions of writing and representation toward more innovative forms, has generated much debate. Anderson (2006), for example has suggested that autoethnography be categorised into either 'analytic' or 'evocative' forms. Other more 'evocatively orientated' autoethnographers (e.g., Ellis & Bochner, 2006) view with suspicion attempts to shift autoethnography away from its more innovative, personally-engaged and emotional forms and back towards what they perceive as more traditional, (neo)realist, ethnographic content and style. As Atkinson (2006, p. 402) reminds us, however: " ... all ethnographic work implies a degree of personal engagement with the field and with the data ... Autoethnography is, it would appear, grounded in an explicit recognition of those biographical and personal foundations." As Ellis, Adams and Bochner (2011) succinctly note, autoethnographers use personal experience to illustrate cultural experience and thus make characteristics of a culture familiar for both insiders and outsiders. Of interest to autoethnographers is the notion of the *ethnós* (Greek for 'race' or 'nation', but nowadays generally extended to include a cultural, subcultural or social group of some kind), which, as Denzin (1983, pp. 133–4) notes, holds its own sets of meanings, structures and normative order. Exactly who constitutes the particular *ethnós* of course is open to debate: who should be included and who excluded? Ty and Verduyn (2008, p. 4) caution against essentialist notions of the social group, and in terms of 'insider' status, interactionists would remind us that membership of any social group or category – our group 'insiderness' – is ever shifting, fluid, mutable and context-dependent. With regard to my own sporting subcultural group membership, for example, I am a non-élite but *serious*, female distance runner. But, further, I am a cross-country specialist rather than a road or track runner. I am a white female in a middle-class professional occupational group. My current distance is nowadays between 5 and 10 miles, which would not constitute 'distance' for many runners. Thus, my group membership is complex, shifting and context-dependent.

In a similar vein and from an anthropological perspective, Strathern (1987), has problematized the 'insider' status of professional anthropologists who portray themselves as members of the culture they study, but who, Strathern notes, do not necessarily hold the same views as do the 'natives'. But, again who are the 'authentic' natives or the 'insiders' to a given culture? It is debatable whether anyone can ever be deemed a 'complete member' of any culture, subculture or social group, for what criteria would have to be fulfilled in order to ascertain complete membership, and for how long does one have to be a member? Who should decide and agree upon such criteria? Perhaps then, it is more accurate to think in terms of a continuum, of degrees of 'insiderness', which change over time, place and social context and bring into interactional play different 'selves' in different contexts, as symbolic interactionists would contend. As an academic sociologist, a veteran, cross-country, female distance runner (amongst many other things), I hold membership of various social groups, but at any one point, my felt membership may relate to any one or combination of these groups, or indeed to none of the above.

Within research on sport and physical culture, autoethnographic researchers have addressed a wide spectrum of different sports and physical cultures, using different representational forms, ranging from highly evo-cative poetic or prose representations (e.g., Stone, 2009 on excessive exercising and anorexia; Denison, 2006 on running), to more 'analytic' representations where sections of autoethnographic narrative are subject to theoretical analysis in a more (neo)realist style (e.g., Allen-Collinson, 2003 on distance running and temporality; McMahon & Dinan Thompson, 2011, on elite swimming and regulation of the body). To date, SPC autoethnographic researchers have in general tended to employ more analytic forms, but the analytic-evocative spectrum (see Anderson, 2006, and Ellis, 1997 for contrasting perspectives) means that the autoethnographic genre is open to a vast range of different styles and usages. As Sparkes (1998, p. 380) notes in relation to more innovative forms of qualitative research in general: "there can be no canonical approach to this form of inquiry, no recipes or rigid formulas." This openness to different forms, and refusal to be pigeonholed, is perhaps one of the great strengths of autoethnographic research. To give just a flavour of this burgeoning field within SPC, some of the sporting and physical cultural contexts and experiences studied to date include triathlon (Drummond, 2010; McCarville, 2007), running (Allen-Collinson & Hockey, 2001; Denison, 2006; Stone, 2009), rugby (Mellick & Fleming, 2010), competitive rowing (Purdy, Potrac, & Jones, 2008; Tsang, 2000), windsurfing (Humberstone, 2011), sports coaching (Jones, 2006, 2009), and performance psychology and dance (Lussier-Ley, 2010), to name just a few domains, which have sparked the interest of SPC researchers. These studies involve a range of different ways of utilising autoethnography and in the next section I consider some of the 'hows' of undertaking a research project using this approach.

DOING AUTOETHNOGRAPHY: RESEARCH DESIGN AND PRACTICE

In this section, to illustrate some of the key methodological elements, I focus upon two particular research studies where an autoethnographic research approach was adopted. The first was a collaborative autoethnography

I undertook some years ago in conjunction with my co-runner and co-researcher, Dr John Hockey, when we were both suffering from long-term knee injuries, and decided to research our experiences. The second was an autoethnographic study of female distance running in public space. I also address below some of the salient ethical issues involved in undertaking these and analogous autoethnographic research projects.

The Collaborative Autoethnographic Project

First, and commensurate with an automethodological approach help contextualise the research discussed here, I provide some background biographical information to the collaborative autoethnographic study[1], much of which is also relevant to the second, solo autoethnographic research project. At the time of the collaborative study, both I and my co-researcher were (and still are) two non-élite, but 'serious' middle/long-distance runners with athletic biographies of distance running and racing, requiring a commitment to training 6 or 7 days a week, sometimes twice daily, for 26 years (author) and 44 years (training partner) respectively. For 17 years we trained together on a regular and frequent basis when living in the same cities. As *veteran* runners, our degree of involvement in running mirrors Stebbins' (1992, p. 6 *et seq.*) concept of 'serious leisure', involving the following elements: perseverance, progressive improvement (generally!), significant personal effort based on specially-acquired knowledge and training, durable benefits (such as health and fitness), a unique ethos or idioculture, and a tendency to identify strongly with the chosen pursuit. All six of these dimensions figured prominently in our running biographies. By strange coincidence, on different days during a particular windswept November week of training in the UK, we both suffered knee injuries, occasioned primarily by having to train in the winter dark on a local park strewn with branches and other assorted débris following several days of storms and high winds. Early in the training week, I stumbled into a branch, twisting my right knee sharply and had to half-run, half-limp through the remaining mileage that evening. Later that same week, my training partner slipped on muddy terrain, wrenching his left knee. It quite quickly became apparent to both of us that the knee injuries were more serious than the usual bodily 'niggles' that frequently plague habitual runners. As a consequence we arrived at a decision systematically to document our experiences, one of our key motives being to extract something positive out of a very negative athletic context. We therefore together designed a

collaborative research study of the injury and subsequent rehabilitative
process; a process that eventually turned out to span a period of around two
years. We decided that a collaborative autoethnographic approach –
sometimes termed 'duoethnography' (Ngunjiri, Hernandez, & Chang, 2010)
combining our own personal experiences as distance runners, would provide
the best research strategy for investigating our individual and joint lived
experiences of the injury process, and providing researcher 'triangulation'
(metaphorically if not literally). Collaborative autoethnography is a wide-
ranging form of autoethnography, spanning the involvement of two co-
researchers/co-authors to construct the narrative, as in this particular case,
to the involvement of many others to produce more of a 'community
autoethnography' (e.g. Toyosaki, Pensoneau-Conway, Wendt, & Leathers,
2009) format, with multiple authorial voices.

Data Collection and Analysis

The data collection process upon which we decided involved the
construction of detailed, individual and collective research logs throughout
the two-year, often painful and distressing, injury and rehabilitative period.
This systematic documentation was a habit already familiar to us, not only
via our academic research work but also as a habitual practice amongst
serious runners, who record their daily performance in training logs. We
were thus used to keeping training logs to record details of timings, dis-
tances, terrain type, weather conditions, health and so on. For the research
project, we replaced these with 'injury-rehabilitation logs', to record
individual and collective engagement with the injured state, and our
attempts to regain sufficient fitness to run again at the level we had enjoyed
previous to incurring the injuries. This data collection was undertaken via
field note books and micro tape recorders, the latter accompanying us on
training sessions, to some physiotherapy sessions, and also throughout the
day for 'head notes' or 'notes to self' when thoughts occurred to us, for
example when travelling to work in the car. We did briefly consider video
recording parts of our training and rehabilitative sessions but quickly
abandoned this idea, deciding it would be too cumbersome to be prac-
ticable, and would interfere too much with the actual training. Audiotapes
were transcribed as soon as possible after recording, usually at weekends. In
addition to our individual research logs, we created a joint analytic log in
which our discussions and salient themes, theoretical ideas and concepts
were recorded. So, for example, if we found that one of us had documented
a particular narrative theme, we would discuss this, posing questions,

challenging each other's assumptions, trying to pinpoint the precise composition of that theme, its boundaries and its connections to other themes already generated either singly or jointly.

As two qualitative sociologists with strong running identities, we shared many similarities, but inevitably also diverged – sometimes radically – in relation to our lived experiences and also our ideas. As part of the data analysis process, within our joint log, thematic or conceptual differences between our individual accounts were identified and, if possible, reconciled. But where no analytical reconciliation proved achievable or indeed desirable, we were content to accept and record the differences. We also discussed the reasons for such divergence and the impact, if any, upon the process of handling our injuries. This added a further analytic dimension to the data collection and analysis process (cf., Ngunjiri et al., 2010). We thus acted as the 'primary recipient' (Ochs & Capps, 1996) of each other's data, discussing events, experiences and interpretations, supplying regular feedback and critique. Subsequently, we analysed and re-analysed our journal entries, primarily via thematic analysis, employing processes of 're-memory' (Sanders-Bustle & Oliver, 2001) to send ourselves back in what we termed our 'time tunnel' to try to recapture as vividly as possible the sometimes wildly oscillating emotions of the injury and rehabilitative journey (Allen-Collinson, 2005).

In this particular form of 'concurrent autoethnography' (Ngunjiri et al., 2010), we moved between individual, divergent activities (e.g., self-reflection, recording our individual logs) and collaborative, convergent activities (e.g., discussions and recording of the joint log) at various points in the research process. Undertaking the collaborative autoethnography fulfilled a range of purposes, including at times the cathartic and therapeutic and, as we had originally hoped, it did generate something positive out of what was a very difficult, painful (psychologically and physically) experience. Indeed, the long-term injury/rehabilitative process, and also the autoethnographic research process itself, proved to be learning and life-changing experiences. They demonstrated both the importance of shared human lived experiences, but also the limits of intersubjectivity – the times of existential loneliness and despair, which even the most experienced, supportive and caring of running life-world inhabitants could not share.

The Autophenomenographic Project

The second autoethnographic and autophenomenographic (see Conclusion) research project was a study of female distance running. In order to document my lived experience of training for middle/long-distance running, I again maintained a research log, in this instance for a period of just over three years, incorporating detailed subjective and corporeal experiences of daily training sessions. The research approach adhered quite closely to Giorgi's (1997) guidelines for undertaking empirical-phenomenological research, and included the following stages: i) the collection of concrete descriptions of phenomena from an insider perspective (i.e., as a female distance runner); ii) initial impressionistic readings of the log entries to gain a feel for the whole; iii) in-depth, close re-reading of these descriptions as part of a process of thorough data-immersion, to identify themes and sub-themes; iv) free imaginative variation, where I searched for the most fundamental meanings of a phenomenon, its 'essential' or core character-istics. This stage of the method involved imaginatively varying elements of any given phenomenon to ascertain whether it remained identifiable after various imagined changes. This assisted in the identification and analysis of 'essences': those elements which were, for me, necessary for the phenomenon to be experienced as that particular phenomenon; and then finally, v) the production of the general account of experience. There were specific challenges in undertaking the solo study, and below I outline one of the classic problems familiar to 'insider' researchers: that of seeking to make the familiar strange and thus bringing the mundane everyday world to heightened analytic attention via a process of 'bracketing'.

In my case, while a relatively long 'career' (in the symbolic interactionist sense, rather than as a professional athlete) provided reassurance regarding the fulfilment of Garfinkel's (2002) 'unique adequacy requirement' for the researcher to have great familiarity with the phenomenon, it also presented somewhat of a problem. The need for familiarity rendered problematic a central element in the phenomenological method, *epoché* or 'bracketing' – the attempted suspension (as far as possible) of the researcher's pre-suppositions and assumptions about a phenomenon – thus requiring heightened reflexivity of me as an autophenomenographic researcher. I should stress that here it is a question of attempting to suspend what Gearing (2004, p. 1443) terms 'internal (researcher) suppositions': my own personal, insider subcultural knowledge of distance running, together with my academic knowledge-theoretical and conceptual for example, and my own personal history and lived experience of being a female distance runner. In order to bracket (in a sociological-phenomenological sense, rather than a more philosophical one) my own preconceptions and taken-for-granted assumptions about female running in public space, in the project I engaged in two bracketing practices aimed at making the familiar strange: (1) discussions with both insiders and non-insiders to the distance-running subculture; and (2) in-depth reading of detailed ethnographic accounts of other sporting activities. This latter was undertaken in order to compare and contrast other sports with my own lived experience of running, including the gendered dimension where this was explicitly analysed, for example in accounts of women's triathlon (Cronan & Scott, 2008; Granskog, 2003) and mountain climbing (Chisholm, 2008). As a female runner who undertakes the vast majority of training in public space, I am well aware that such space is also gendered, as feminist analysts have long identified. My running in public space is thus lived and felt at the individual, subjective level, but is also profoundly structurally shaped by my own socio-cultural (and subcultural) and historical location.

Ethical Dimensions of Autoethnography

At this point, it is worth discussing generally some of the oft-overlooked ethical dimensions of undertaking autoethnographic research, whether individual or collaborative. Although writing about our own sporting and/ or physical cultural experiences may initially appear to be relatively devoid of ethical concerns, when compared with other forms of research with human participants, ethical issues and dilemmas certainly arise for auto-ethnographers. While we are often accustomed to considering carefully the protection of our research participants, autoethnographers do not always devote the same attention to protecting themselves in the research process, should this prove necessary. Indeed, actually engaging in the autoethno-graphic process itself can constitute an emotionally painful and potentially self-injurious act. Chatham-Carpenter (2010), for example, describes vividly how, during the writing of her autoethnography of anorexia, she experi-enced the compulsion to publish her work become intertwined with the compulsion of her anorexia. Furthermore, there arises the question of how far along the self-disclosure/exposure and vulnerability route the auto-ethnographer wishes to locate her/himself, and how honest s/he chooses to be in creating and representing the self. Autoethnography can confront us with acute dilemmas regarding our presentation of self (Goffman, 1974), and just how much sensitive biographical information to reveal. As Ellis (1999) notes, the autoethnographer makes her/himself vulnerable in reveal-ing sensitive, intimate information, and subsequently being unable to retract this, having no control over how readers might interpret sensitive bio-graphical information. Writing in a personalised and often emotional, open and vulnerable style, challenges the widely held orthodoxy of researcher as neutral, objective, coolly rational, and textually absent. This can leave the autoethnographic researcher highly vulnerable to charges of being "irrational, particularistic, private, and subjective, rather than reasonable, universal, public, and objective" (Greenhalgh, 2001, p. 55). Behar (1997, p. 13–14) reminds us of the dangers of over-exposure of the vulnerable self and the need for self-discipline: "Vulnerability doesn't mean that anything personal goes'; the exposure of the self 'has to be essential to the argument, not a decorative flourish, not exposure for its own sake."

A further ethical issue with which autoethnographers contend is that however personal the autoethnography may be, it is likely to feature other social actors with whom the researcher has some degree of relationship or at least of social interaction. As Erben (1993) notes, in his case in relation to autobiography, it is a very rare account that does not contain many – whether shorter or longer – biographies of other people who figure in the writer's life, and thus contribute to the life story being portrayed. In this vein, Wall (2008) highlights some of the dilemmas and difficult judgements arising from recounting her own story of parenting an adopted child. These dilemmas are neatly encapsulated in a footnote where she (2008, p. 51) acknowledges that while she speaks of the autoethnography as 'my' story, her husband and children are also in various ways authors of the story.

Autoethnographers have thus to consider carefully how (and indeed if) certain others are included and represented within the write-up of the research. Even when others are anonymised within the account, at least in terms of remaining formally unnamed, they may nevertheless be identifiable via distinctive social or physical characteristics. Within the field of SPC, Mellick and Fleming (2010) address the ethics of disclosure in relation to a personal narrative that included the portrayal of a particular rugby player with an identifiable biography, which made him a 'unique case study', despite all efforts at anonymisation. The specific ethical dilemma confronting the authors was that the biographical information and international reputation of the player were essential to the theoretical framing of the narrative. Removing this information would have greatly weakened the analysis, and rendered it impotent, in their terms.

Additionally, in relation to the representation of others, there are questions of how exactly to use another person's life to tell our own stories, as Wall (2008: 49) discusses. In the kind of collaborative autoethnographic research project described above, it is standard practice to check and agree with one's co-researcher/author what should be included in (and excluded from) the research write-up; a decision that may require careful negotiation.

Fortunately, my co-researcher and I found we shared similar perspectives on the inclusion of more private and sensitive autoethnographic data. Securing this form of consent from other participants in an autoethnographic project, however incidental to the account, may not prove quite so straightforward or indeed even possible. In our collaborative autoethnography, photographs of others were included in published articles based on the study. Although it would have been difficult to ascertain the identity of any individual, given that the photographs were taken at some distance, identification may just have been possible for someone familiar with the individuals portrayed. Similarly, in the accounts generated from the autoethnographic data, family members, friends and others could – with some detective work – have been identifiable.

A final ethics-related point I highlight here concerns the wish not to finalise the stories of other co-authors and co-participants in one's autoethnographic narrative, but to engage in dialogical rather than monological research (see Smith, Allen-Collinson, Phoenix, Brown, & Sparkes, 2009). This means having a willingness to converse with others and indeed with the autoethnographic process itself (cf., Wall, 2008: 40), rather than seeking to give 'the final word' on events. To this end, autoethnographers often deliberately employ relational language to create and promote reader-author dialogue, rather than making monologic pronouncements. To explain briefly, for Bakhtin (1984) and Frank (2004), monologue is a form of self-narrative that purports to be self-sufficient, telling what the author or speaker knows and to what the listener must attend and learn from. Bakhtin's (1984) conceptualisaton of monologue portrays a self-narrative seeking, explicitly or implicitly, to *merge* with the other, to assimilate others into the narrator's self, via the abridging of difference and distance. According to Bakhtin (1984), dialogical writing involves abandoning the illusion that we can, even with the best of intentions, merge with another person. To act ethically, we should never presume to know exactly how another person feels, and speak *for* them. Instead, we should acknowledge and respect alterity and seek to preserve some intersubjective distance. Critical reflexivity is crucial for the autoethnographer, as indeed for qualitative researchers in general, who must guard against *merging* with other participants, however much of the ethnographic field we feel we hold in common. An important consequence for this form of research is that no individual autoethnographer's story is completely and entirely her/his own; the voices and selves of others intertwine with ourselves and our stories, as Wall (2008) perceptively highlights in her autoethnographic study of adoptive parenting.

KEY FINDINGS OF THE STUDIES

The purpose of the collaborative autoethnographic study was to analyse the impact of relatively severe and chronic injuries on our identities as two amateur, non-élite, but *serious* and long-term middle/long-distance runners, and to explore the rehabilitative journey back to (what we hoped would be) full running fitness. In analysing the considerable amount of data generated by the methods portrayed above, we found several key themes emerged, several of which I portray here. We had both agreed when undertaking the research, that while we would certainly publish jointly off the data, each of us would also be free to undertake his and her own separate analysis and write-up, and to publish individually from the project. One of the key themes, which we identified jointly, cohered strongly with the symbolic interactionist concept of identity work. Such identity work, it emerged, played a major role in providing continuity of identity during the liminality of long-term injury and rehabilitation, and the 'injury time' that posed a fundamental challenge to our athletic identities. In our subsequent analyses and reports of the study, we employed Snow and Anderson's (1995) and also Perinbanayagam's (2000) interactionist theoretical conceptualisations in order to examine the various forms of identity work in which we engaged (for more details, see Allen-Collinson & Hockey, 2007). Identity work has been defined as:

> ... the range of activities individuals engage in to create, present and sustain personal
> identities that are congruent with and supportive of the self-concept. So defined, identity
> work may involve a number of complementary activities: a) arrangement of physical
> settings or props; b) cosmetic face-work or the arrangement of personal appearance; c)
> selective association with other individuals and groups; d) verbal constructions and
> assertion of personal identities (Snow & Anderson, 1995, p. 241).

In Perinbanayagam's (2000) categorisation, these activities are reformulated as *materialistic, associative* and *vocabularic* identifications respectively, and these and Snow & Anderson's categories were found to be highly applicable to the identity work we undertook as (temporarily) non-running runners. Such 'work' was found to be central, and indeed crucial, in sustaining credible athletic identities in the face of intense disruption to the running self, and also in generating momentum towards the goal of restitution to full running fitness; a goal eventually achieved after a two-year journey.

A second key finding for me was the temporal dimension of the injury and rehabilitation process; a theme which at the time of writing was found to be under-explored within SPC studies. Despite a growing corpus of research on the sociology of time, and with some notable exceptions (e.g., Eichberg, 1982) relatively little sports literature had taken time as its analytic focus. This seemed to me a curious lacuna, particularly given the centrality of time within most sports, and certainly within running, where race times, personal bests, and so on are salient features of the sporting context. As Adam (2000) notes, there is still a propensity for social time to be taken-for-granted, left unproblematised and treated by many social science researchers as a neutral medium within which events simply take place. From the autoethnographic data, four categories of time emerged strongly: linear, cyclical, inner and biographical time (see Allen-Collinson, 2003). One of the main findings was the need for sports coaches, physiotherapists and other health-care practitioners involved with injured sportspeople, to take into account the subjective, 'inner-time' (*durée*), dimension of injury and rehabilitative processes, in order better to tailor effective individual treatment plans.

CONCLUSION

In sum, autoethnographers seek to connect the personal to the (sub)cultural, often writing in highly evocative and personal ways, and thus, for those working from a more traditional perspective, transgressing orthodox requirements for social science research. The autoethnographic genre often boldly traverses and blurs distinctions of the personal and the social, and of self and other. For many of us who have tried working with this relatively novel research approach, autoethnography has certain strengths. These include its openness to new directions and multiple forms, its wide-ranging, protean nature, and its refusal to be tied down and tightly constrained by adherence to traditional notions of validity and other inappropriate positivistic judgment criteria. The evocative and more literary writing styles often offer striking and thought-provoking ways of addressing mundane experience and subjecting it to rigorous analysis. The 'insider' perspective gives autoethnographers the advantage of access to in-depth and often highly nuanced meanings, knowledge about, and lived experience of the field of study. This brings into play a wide range of resources, which would not normally be available to 'outsider' researchers. In inviting the reader to share the feelings and the sensations, and to connect with the author's experience, autoethnographers often write highly readable, insightful and thought-provoking work, vividly bringing alive sub/cultural experiences for those unfamiliar with the social terrain under study. Further, the requirement for the researcher explicitly to situate and analyse her/himself in the dual role of researcher and participant means that the reader is enabled to make some kind of judgment about the author's legitimacy with regard to portraying and interpreting the specific social context studied.

In terms of weaknesses, autoethnography in general has been accused of a lack of academic rigour, of self-indulgence and navel-gazing, and employing a diarist style, particularly when more evocative forms are, erroneously, believed to be representative of what is a highly diverse and multi-stranded field. For those seeking to adhere to the traditional triad of evaluation criteria appropriate to the scientific method – validity, reliability and generalisability – autoethnographic research would not provide a suitable methodology, and indeed has no concern with fulfilling these criteria. The kinds of assessment criteria posited for autoethnographic – and also much ethnographic – work, are wide-ranging, and generally acknowledge the relativism of 'truth' and knowledge claims as being dependent upon historical and socio-cultural context. Alternative criteria suggested for assessing auto/ethnographic research include concepts such as *credibility* and *verisimilitude*. Richardson (2000, p. 254), for example, argues in relation to ethnography that it should express a reality that 'seems true', furnishing us with a "credible account of a cultural, social, individual, or communal sense of the "real""; a sentiment that also holds in relation to good autoethnography, many of us would argue. A further judgment criterion highlighted as important is the notion of *resonance*, where the research findings and write-up should reverberate with the experience of the reader so that s/he can identify at some level with what is being communicated, and also feel empathy for the author/researcher, thus achieving what Dadds (2008) terms 'empathetic validity'.

It should be remembered, however, that while autoethnographic research certainly does incorporate very personal, evocative and poetic accounts, seeking to promote empathetic understanding, it also includes highly analytic and theoretical work under its wide *aegis*. It makes little sense to evaluate both forms, located at different ends of the analytic-evocative spectrum, via the same criteria. Furthermore, as Sparkes and Smith (2009) argue in relation to judging qualitative research in general, evaluation criteria should never be viewed as fixed and universal, but rather as open to reinterpretation as times, conditions and research purposes change. Thus, in order to be fair and ethical, they argue, we need to adopt a mode of connoisseurship in order to make judgments vis-à-vis different kinds of research. One set of evaluation criteria most certainly does not fit all.

With regard to future directions, one of the strengths of autoethnography is its openness to new uses and formats, and I think that a new form of the genre, 'autophenomenography' (Allen-Collinson, 2011a, 2011b; Gruppetta, 2004) holds rich possibilities for SPC researchers. In this form of research, as described above in relation to the autophenomenographic study of female distance running, the primary focus is upon the researcher's lived experience of a phenomenon or phenomena rather than upon her or his cultural or subcultural location. This latter is more usually the locus of scholarly attention in autoethnography, although clearly cultural location and lived experience are closely inter-twined, certainly in the application of phenomenology by SPC researchers in the social sciences, rather than in its 'purer' philosophical form. In autophenomenography, the self is engaged in a specific way: in relation to phenomena, or things as they appear to the conscious mind. This is a research approach that I found interesting but also very challenging in relation to my own lived body experiences of distance running. I should explain that I choose to use the term autophenomenography rather than autophenomenology here for two reasons. First, as with autoethnography, 'graphy' is taken as applicable to the research process in general as well as to the written, or representational product of that process. Second, autophenomenology has specific and highly contested meanings within phenomenology (e.g., Drummond, 2007) and here is not really the forum to engage in such debates.

Although Gruppetta (2004) is the first person (to my knowledge) to make reference to autophenomenography, she does not go into any detail regarding how actually to utilize this approach, and it would seem to offer exciting possibilities to add to the developing corpus of autoethnographic work. I have suggested above using a form of Giorgi's empirical phenomenology to undertake autophenomenography, but others may have different ideas as to how profitably to engage in this form of research; the way is open! Analogous to its autoethnographic sibling, autophenomenography is capable of producing the rich, finely textured, 'thick descriptions' of first-person experience, and bringing to life the felt, lived, corporeal experience, so central to much of our participation in sport and physical cultures. Within the autophenomenographic genre too there is scope for a wide spectrum of representational styles, including evocative forms such as poetic representations and performative, audience-interactive presentations, already familiar to those of us working with autoethnography. Along with the use of collaborative and community autoethnographies, I envisage autophenomenography to be one of the key new directions for those employing 'auto-methodology' (Pensoneau-Conway & Toyosaki, 2011) within SPC.

This chapter has considered autoethnography as a relatively novel research approach within SPC, one which offers a variety of modes of engaging with self, or perhaps more accurately, selves – to reflect the context-dependency of our felt identities. Whilst autoethnography undoubtedly has proved a vibrant and innovative research approach for those working in SPC (and beyond), there are both strengths and weaknesses as delineated above. The key task, as with any form of research, is to decide what methodological approach will best suit the ontological and epistemological bases, and the aims and objectives of the particular research study. Autoethnographic research offers, I would argue, a means of gaining rich and nuanced insights into personal lived experience and situating these within a wider socio-cultural context; insights which are unlikely to be accessible via more 'orthodox' research approaches. It thus adds a potent additional element to the methodological pantheon available to us as researchers in SPC.

FIVE KEY READINGS

1. Allen-Collinson, J. & Hockey, J. (2005). Autoethnography: Self-indulgence or rigorous methodology? In M. J. McNamee (Ed.), *Philosophy and the Sciences of Exercise, Health and Sport: Critical Perspectives on Research Methods*. London: Routledge, pp. 187–202.
This chapter sets out the ways in which autoethnography has been and can be utilised within research in sport, exercise and health sciences, also addressing head-on criticisms of the approach as 'self-indulgent' and narcissistic.

2. Anderson, L. (2006). Analytic autoethnography. *Journal of Contemporary Ethnography*, *35*(4), 373–395.
This article argues (not uncontentiously) for a distinction between 'analytic' and more 'evocative' forms of autoethnography, and posits that the former refers to research in which the researcher is: a full member in the research group or setting, visible as such in published texts, and committed to developing theoretical understandings.

3. Ellis, C. & Bochner, A. P. (2000). Autoethnography, personal narrative, reflexivity. In N. K. Denzin & Y. S. Lincoln (Eds.), *Handbook of Qualitative Research* (2nd ed.). Thousand Oaks, CA: Sage.
This chapter considers, among other things, issues of representation and autoethnographic writing as a method of inquiry that requires great

reflexivity, and takes the author on a journey through various stages of self-reflection.

4. Jones, R. (2006). Dilemmas, maintaining 'face' and paranoia: An average coaching life. *Qualitative Inquiry, 12*(5), 1012–1021.
This is an interesting and highly readable example of an article that combines evocative and analytic autoethnography by presenting the evocative narrative of the author himself (as a coach of a semi-professional soccer team) as the core of the article, with the theoretical and analytic section provided in the form of end notes.

5. Reed-Danahay, D. (Ed.) (1997). *Auto/Ethnography: Rewriting the self and the social.* Oxford: Berg.
A 'classic', original introduction to autoethnography.

NOTE

1. My co-researcher has kindly given his consent for a little of his biographical information to be included for the purposes of this chapter.

REFERENCES

Adam, B. (2000). The temporal gaze: The challenge for social theory in the context of GM Food. *British Journal of Sociology, 5*, 125–142.

Allen-Collinson, J. (2003). Running into injury time: Distance running and temporality. *Sociology of Sport Journal, 20*(4), 331–350.

Allen-Collinson, J. (2005). Emotions, interaction and the injured sporting body. *International Review for the Sociology of Sport, 40*(2), 221–240.

Allen-Collinson, J. (2011a). Intention and epochē in tension: Autophenomenography, bracketing and a novel approach to researching sporting embodiment. *Qualitative Research in Sport, Exercise & Health, 3*(1), 48–62.

Allen-Collinson, J. (2011b). Feminist phenomenology and the woman in the running body. *Sport, Ethics & Philosophy, 5*(3), 287–302.

Allen-Collinson, J., & Hockey, J. (2001). Runners' tales: Autoethnography, injury and narrative. *Auto/Biography, IX*(1 & 2), 95–106.

Allen-Collinson, J., & Hockey, J. (2007). 'Working out' identity: Distance runners and the management of disrupted identity. *Leisure Studies, 26*(4), 381–398.

Anderson, L. (2006). Analytic autoethnography. *Journal of Contemporary Ethnography, 35*(4), 373–395.

Atkinson, P. (2006). Rescuing autoethnography. *Journal of Contemporary Ethnography, 35*(4), 400–404.

Bakhtin, M. (1984). *Problems of Dostoevsky's poetics (translated and edited by C. Emerson)*. Minneapolis: University of Minnesota Press.

Behar, R. (1997). *The vulnerable observer: Anthropology that breaks your heart*. Boston: Beacon.

Chatham-Carpenter, A. (2010). 'Do thyself no harm': Protecting ourselves as autoethnographers. *Journal of Research Practice*, 6(1), Article M1. Retrieved from http://jrp.icaap.org/index.php/jrp/article/view/213/183. Accessed 9 August 2012.

Chisholm, D. (2008). Climbing like a girl: An exemplary adventure in feminist phenomenology. *Hypatia*, 23(1), 9–40.

Cronan, M. K., & Scott, D. (2008). Triathlon and women's narratives of bodies and sport. *Leisure Sciences*, 30, 17–34.

Dadds, M. (2008). Empathetic validity in practitioner research. *Educational Action Research*, 16(2), 279–290.

Denison, J. (2006). The way we ran. Reimagining research and the self. *Journal of Sport and Social Issues*, 30(4), 333–339.

Denzin, N. K. (1983). Interpretative interactionism. In G. Morgan (Ed.), *Beyond method: Strategies for social research* (pp. 129–146). Beverley Hills, CA: Sage.

Denzin, N. K., & Lincoln, Y. S. (2000). The policies and practices of interpretation. In N. K. Denzin & Y. S. Lincoln (Eds.), *Handbook of qualitative research* (2nd ed., pp. 897–992). Thousand Oaks, CA: Sage.

Drummond, J. J. (2007). Phenomenology: Neither auto- nor hetero- be. *Phenomenology and the Cognitive Sciences*, 6, 57–74.

Drummond, M. (2010). The natural: An autoethnography of a masculinized body in sport. *Men and Masculinities*, 12(3), 374–389.

Eichberg, H. (1982). Stopwatch, horizontal bar, gymnasium: The technology of sports in the 18th and 19th centuries. *Journal of the Philosophy of Sport*, 9(1), 43–59.

Ellis, C. (1997). Evocative autoethnography. In W. Tierney & Y. Lincoln (Eds.), *Representation and the text* (pp. 115–139). New York: State University of New York Press.

Ellis, C. (1999). Heartful autoethnography. *Qualitative Health Research*, 9(5), 669–683.

Ellis, C., Adams, T. E., & Bochner, A. (2011). Autoethnography: An overview. *Forum: Qualitative Social Research/Sozialforschung*, 12(1), Article 10. Retrieved from http://www.qualitative-research.net/index.php/fqs/article/viewArticle/1589/3095. Accessed 9 August 2012.

Ellis, C., & Bochner, A. (2006). Analyzing analytic autoethnography: An autopsy. *Journal of Contemporary Ethnography*, 35(4), 429–449.

Ellis, C., & Bochner, A. P. (Eds.). (1996). *Composing ethnography: Alternative forms of qualitative writing*. Walnut Creek, CA: Alta Mira Press.

Ellis, C., & Bochner, A. P. (2000). Autoethnography, personal narrative, reflexivity. In N. K.Denzin & Y. S. Lincoln (Eds.), *Handbook of qualitative research* (2nd ed., pp. 733–768). Thousand Oaks, CA: Sage.

Erben, M. (1993). The problem of other lives: Social perspectives on written biography. *Sociology*, 27(1), 15–25.

Fiske, J. (1990). Ethnosemiotics: Some personal and theoretical reflections. *Cultural Studies*, 4, 85–99.

Frank, A. (2004). *The renewal of generosity*. Chicago: The University of Chicago Press.

Garfinkel, H. (2002). *Ethnomethodology's program: Working out Durkheim's aphorism*. New York: Rowman & Littlefield.

Gearing, R. E. (2004). Bracketing in research: A typology. *Qualitative Health Research, 14*(10), 1429–1452.

Giorgi, A. P. (1997). The theory, practice and evaluation of the phenomenological method as a qualitative research procedure. *Journal of Phenomenological Psychology, 28*(2), 235–260.

Goffman, E. (1974). *The presentation of self in everyday life.* Harmondsworth: Penguin

Granskog, J. (2003). Just 'Tri' and 'Du' it: The variable impact of female involvement in the triathlon/duathlon sport culture. In A. Bolin & J. Granskog (Eds.), *Athletic intruders. Ethnographic research on women, culture, and exercise* (pp. 27–52). New York: State University of New York Press.

Greenhalgh, S. (2001). *Under the medical gaze: Facts and fictions of chronic pain.* Berkeley: University of California Press.

Gruppetta, M. (2004). Autophenomenography? Alternative uses of autobiographically based research. In P. L. Jeffery (Ed.), *Association for Active Researchers in Education (AARE) Conference Paper Abstracts – 2004.* Sydney: AARE. Retrieved from http://www.aare. edu.au/04pap/gru04228.pdf

Humberstone, B. (2011). Embodiment and social and environmental action in nature-based sport: Spiritual spaces. *Leisure Studies, 30*(4), 495–512.

Jones, R. L. (2006). Dilemmas, maintaining 'face' and paranoia: An average coaching life. *Qualitative Inquiry, 12*(5), 1012–1021.

Jones, R. L. (2009). Coaching as caring (the smiling gallery): Accessing hidden knowledge. *Physical Education and Sport Pedagogy, 14*(4), 377–390.

Lussier-Ley, C. (2010). Dialoguing with body: A self study in relational pedagogy through embodiment and the therapeutic relationship. *The Qualitative Report, 15*(1), 197–214.

McCarville, R. (2007). From a fall in the mall to a run in the sun: One journey to Ironman triathlon. *Leisure Sciences, 29*, 159–173.

McMahon, J., & Dinan Thompson, M. (2011). 'Body work regulation of a swimmer body': An autoethnography from an Australian élite swimmer. *Sport, Education and Society, 16*(1), 35–50.

Mellick, M., & Fleming, S. (2010). Personal narrative and the ethics of disclosure: A case study from élite sport. *Qualitative Research, 10*(3), 299–314.

Ngunjiri, F.W., Hernandez, K.-A. C., & Chang, H. (2010). Living autoethnography: Connecting life and research. *Journal of Research Practice, 6*(1), Article E1. Retrieved from http://jrp.icaap.org/index.php/jrp/article/viewArticle/241/186

Ochs, E., & Capps, L. (1996). Narrating the self. *Annual Review of Anthropology, 25*, 19–43.

Pensoneau-Conway, S. L., & Toyosaki, S. (2011). Autoethodology: Tracing a home for praxis-oriented ethnography. *International Journal of Qualitative Methods, 10*(4), 378–399.

Perinbanayagam, R. S. (2000). *The presence of self.* Oxford: Rowman & Littlefield.

Purdy, L., Potrac, P., & Jones, R. L. (2008). Power, consent and resistance: An autoethnography of competitive rowing. *Sport, Education and Society, 13*(3), 319–336.

Reed-Danahay, D. (Ed.). (1997). *Auto/Ethnography. Rewriting the self and the social.* Oxford: Berg.

Richardson, L. (1994). Writing: A method of inquiry. In N. K. Denzin & Y. S. Lincoln (Eds.), *Handbook of qualitative research* (pp. 516–529). London: Sage.

Richardson, L. (2000). Evaluating ethnography. *Qualitative Inquiry, 6*, 253–256.

Sanders-Bustle, L., & Oliver, K. L. (2001). The role of physical activity in the lives of researchers: A body-narrative. *Studies in Philosophy and Education, 20*, 507–520.

212   JACQUELYN ALLEN-COLLINSON

Smith, B., Allen-Collinson, J., Phoenix, C., Brown, D., & Sparkes, A. (2009). Dialogue, monologue, and boundary crossing within research encounters: A performative narrative analysis. *International Journal of Sport & Exercise Psychology*, 7(3), 342–359.

Snow, D. A., & Anderson, L. (1995). The problem of identity construction among the homeless. In N. J. Hermann & L. T. Reynolds (Eds.), *Symbolic interaction: An introduction to social psychology*. New York: General Hall, Inc.

Sparkes, A. C. (1998). Validity in qualitative inquiry and the problem of criteria: Implications for sport psychology. *The Sport Psychologist*, 12, 363–386.

Sparkes, A. C., & Smith, B. (2009). Judging the quality of qualitative inquiry: Criteriology and relativism in action. *Psychology of Sport and Exercise*, 10, 491–497.

Spry, T. (2001). Performing autoethnography: An embodied methodological praxis. *Qualitative Inquiry*, 7(6), 706–732.

Stebbins, R. A. (1992). *Amateurs, professionals and serious leisure*. Montréal & Kingston: McGill-Queen's University Press.

Strathern, M. (1987). The limits of auto-anthropology. In A. Jackson (Ed.), *Anthropology at home* (pp. 16–37). London: Tavistock Publications.

Stone, B. (2009). Running man. *Qualitative Research in Sport and Exercise*, 1(1), 67–71.

Tedlock, B. (1991). From participant observation to the observation of participation: The emergence of narrative ethnography. *Journal of Anthropological Research*, 47(1), 69–94.

Toyosaki, S., Pensoneau-Conway, S. L., Wendt, N. A., & Leathers, K. (2009). Community autoethnography: Compiling the personal and resituating whiteness. *Cultural Studies/Critical Methodologies*, 9(1), 56–83.

Tsang, T. (2000). Let me tell you a story: A narrative exploration of identity in high-performance sport. *Sociology of Sport Journal*, 17(1), 44–59.

Ty, E., & Verduyn, C. (2008). *Asian Canadian writing beyond autoethnography*. Waterloo: Wilfrid Laurier Press.

Wall, S. (2008). Easier said than done: Writing an autoethnography. *International Journal of Qualitative Methods*, 7(1), 38–53.

CHAPTER 10

TWO (OR MORE) FEET ARE BETTER THAN ONE: MIXED METHODS RESEARCH IN SPORT AND PHYSICAL CULTURE

Kass Gibson

ABSTRACT

Purpose – *The chapter outlines mixed methods as a recursive and co-operative approach to research. In doing so, it challenges the dominant conception of 'real' mixed methods research as requiring the use of methods from both qualitative and quantitative frameworks by outlining not only logistic and pragmatic issues requiring the attention of researchers but also the underlying philosophical tensions inherent in mixed method designs.*

Design/methodology/approach – *The process of designing a mixed methods project that investigated the sociological and phenomenological impact of running shoes is outlined with reference to the various pragmatic and epistemological considerations of the project.*

Findings – *Many researchers require mixed methods to draw on both quantitative and qualitative techniques. However, this chapter demonstrates that such an understanding of mixed methods marginalises critical*

Qualitative Research on Sport and Physical Culture
Research in the Sociology of Sport, Volume 6, 213–232
Copyright © 2012 by Emerald Group Publishing Limited
All rights of reproduction in any form reserved
ISSN: 1476-2854/doi:10.1108/S1476-2854(2012)0000006013

and interpretivist techniques. It is argued that studies of sport and physical culture have frequently used more than one research method. However, in order for these to be considered mixed methods *studies, an explicit attempt is required to connect each technique of data collection and analysis, regardless of the research paradigm in which they operate.*

Research limitations/implications – *The limitations of mixed methods designs are discussed in relation to pragmatic and logistic concerns as well as the difficulty of connecting methods that present different underlying philosophical assumptions.*

Originality/value – *This chapter demonstrates the design of a mixed methods project from the initial process of identifying a research problem through to data collection, analysis and publication.*

Keywords: Mixed methods; techno-science; running shoes; quantitative research; qualitative research

INTRODUCTION: FIRST STEPS AND MIXED METHODOLOGICAL BEGINNINGS

Upon arriving in Leicestershire, a landlocked and relatively low-lying region of England, in order to attend graduate school, I quickly realised that most of my usual physical recreational activities were no longer viable due to geographical constraints. However, the East Midlands possesses, in abundance, rolling green hills criss-crossed with brooks and forests, populated with birds, badgers and deer, all connected through an expansive network of trails. I ran a lot in high school as additional training and conditioning for my competitive sporting endeavours, and some of my fondest training memories are of early morning runs up the Port Hills behind my family home. As such, I decided that running would be an excellent way to keep active, 'blow out' the proverbial cobwebs before or after the long hours spent in the library stacks, and make the most of my new found home. Best of all for a graduate student, despite the initial outlay for some shoes, running was (and is) free!

Conventional running wisdom stipulates that a high-quality pair of running shoes is required for anyone who is remotely serious about running. Convinced by this subcultural maxim and secure in my biomechanical knowledge, I went to a specialist running store, where I picked up on a peculiar practice. When buying shoes, I usually think about whether I like the colour and shape, as well as whether I have got the right clothes to complement the shoes. In this way, it is a very subjective experience. Purchasing running shoes is quite different – I did not choose a pair of running shoes; I was *prescribed* a pair. It was at that point, in that store, I became interested in the sociological and phenomenological impact of running shoe technology, which became the basis of my research project.

During my undergraduate years, I had a fondness for biomechanics, as well as physical cultural studies. Therefore, the initial attraction of my idea was its ability to incorporate both of these fields. From its earliest days, then, I wanted this project to be structured by a mixed methods design. My desire to interweave these two fields in this particular project reflects the relevance of mixed methods design to research regarding sport and physical culture (SPC). More generally, the study of SPC presents a complex and nuanced nexus of social, cultural and political values and constraints in which people, in all their physical, cognitive, affective and existential dimensions, participate. Accessing and analysing discrete aspects of this nexus, as well as understanding their interconnectedness, logically requires more than one method and type of data. Hence, mixed methods somewhat naturally lend itself to SPC research.

Indeed, many researchers of SPC demonstrate implicit mixed methodological leanings. Certainly, from their very beginning, anthropological studies of the cultural significance of games and play (Geertz, 1973; Gmelch, 1978) and sociological studies of deviance (Polsky, 1967) and sporting cultures (Scott, 1968) all deployed a range of techniques to gather data. This continues today, as evidenced, for example, by studies of 'lifestyle sports' (Stranger, 2011) gendered and gendering processes in SPC (Woodward, 2009), the relationship between environmental politics, sport and physical culture (Collins, 2011), and the media (John & Jackson, 2010).

However, arguably it is in the area of behavioural and psychological research of SPC where mixed methods figures most prominently. This stems mostly from studies addressing adherence to exercise and intervention program evaluation (e.g. Besculides, Zaveri, Farris, & Will, 2006); Fortier et al., 2007; Tjomsland, 2010). One of the key differences between these psychosocial and behavioural studies and the aforementioned sociological and anthropological research is that the former actively identifies itself (at least ostensibly) as mixed method designs vis-à-vis the use of both quantitative and qualitative techniques; whereas the latter are (like my study) mostly rooted in ethnographic methods and supplemented by other techniques, usually interviewing. The embracing of the mixed method label by behavioural and psychosocial research is understandable given the development of mixed methods research.

Mixed methods research history is often traced back to the 'Hawthorne' study of Roethlisberger and Dickson (1939) who, during an experimental project on the effect of illumination levels on worker productivity, discovered that productivity increased when the researchers increased the level of lighting, but productivity failed to decline when the light level decreased. In effect, the experimental variable (illumination) had less of an impact on productivity than the presence of, and surveillance by, researchers. Following this study, a larger project, composed of three phases, was established to understand and explain what had happened in the initial experiment. This involved further field experiments, as well as interviews, in order to untangle what the researchers described as 'a system of interdependent elements' (Roethlisberger & Dickson, 1939, p. 183). Lynd and Lynd's (1927) 'Yankee City' study of social life in the United States undertaken to better understand social institutions, social stratification and social class is also heralded as a groundbreaking mixed methods study.

While many argue that socio-cultural and psychosocial analyses have consistently demonstrated mixed methodological leanings, alluded to in the aforementioned studies of SPC, it was not until the 1970s that explicit mixed methods designs began to gain popularity. Such studies were primarily designed as a process of triangulation whereby 'reliability' and 'validity' (and, therefore, credibility) of research findings are increased through the use of more than one data source or method. Denzin (1978) dubbed the latter approach 'methodological triangulation', where the purpose was to guard again weaknesses of each individual method. Fuelled by emerging critical scholarship, debate raged as to whether qualitative and quantitative data were compatible. Critical scholars debunked of notions of detached, objective researchers highlighting the contextual nature of research, and the value-laden position of the researcher and their choice of theory, methods and subject nature. Miles and Huberman (1994) proposed a solution to bridge the divide evident in the so-called qualitative and quantitative paradigm wars in terms of 'qualitised' (quantitative data converted to narrative) and 'quantitised' (qualitative data converted to numbers). Evidently, the inherent methodological tension between qualitative and quantitative approaches comes to the fore in mixed methods research.

The inherent contradiction between qualitative and quantitative paradigms has led to some questioning of what mixed methods research actually is, what it can be and even if it is really possible. Those who define themselves as 'mixed methodologists', such as Teddlie and Tashakkori (2010), argue that mixed methods must cross paradigmatic boundaries. Such a position is centred on an underlying belief that the use of both qualitative and quantitative methods produces the best of both methodological worlds. Building from this, the inclusion of multiple methods to answer a particular research question, it is argued, will thus create more credible (meaning, triangulated and therefore empirically 'deeper') results. Such arguments are intuitively appealing to empiricists, although critics of the multi-method approach regularly point to the epistemic and ontological divides separating (and potentially irrevocably) subjectivist approaches to objectivist deductive frameworks.

Such an understanding of mixed methods often revolves around quantitative data to support, or more accurately 'bolster', claims made through qualitative research or the use of qualitative data to explicate mediating variables in quantitative studies. This, in effect, reduces both paradigms to caricatures where qualitative research provides the 'whys' and quantitative research the 'whats' and, at a deeper level, continues to privilege the postpositivist scientific tradition concomitantly marginalising critical and interpretative methods.

WALKING THE LINE: BALANCING METHODOLOGICAL CONTRADICTIONS

Pragmatic guides to undertaking research will often gloss over ontological and epistemological issues in their discussions and instructions for conducting research. While such considerations, I think, are of vital importance to any serious researcher, I am sympathetic to their desire to avoid such discussions as much of the philosophical posturing is far removed from the experience of being in the field. However, as you can see from the debates and tensions outline above, one cannot avoid serious consideration of epistemology and ontology when designing and undertaking mixed methods research, especially when deploying methods from either side of the paradigmatic divide.

Those who advocate using mixed methods that cross the paradigmatic divide justify their approach, philosophically, through appeals to the paradigm of pragmatism or multiple paradigm theses (e.g. Teddlie & Tashakkori, 2010). The central argument of such an approach is that philosophical assumptions are conceptual tools and should not take precedent over the practical considerations. The logistical and material issues, not epistemological and ontological debates, should occupy the mind of the researcher, thereby not just skirting around any sound philosophical rationale for the use of different methods but actively dismissing it.

It should be clear to any critical thinker that such an approach does not reflect the 'reality' of the research process but, rather, the contested political and philosophical frontlines of the academy. Not only can the so-called pragmatic approach ensure internal paradigmatic consistency it also reflects the vested ideological interests of certain researchers. Indeed, Green, Kreider, and Mayer (2011) note the untenable nature of the pragmatists' approach, noting our 'methods are indeed framed by the philosophical world-view of the inquirer' (p. 261). Further, Giddings (2006), a self-declared ardent supporter of mixed methods research, warns mixed methodologists against denying the philosophical underpinnings of their research. Giddings (2006, p. 195) pejoratively refers to mixed methods research that fails to address epistemological and ontological considerations as 'positivism dressed in drag' where, 'mixed methods covers for the continuing hegemony of positivism, albeit in its more moderate, post-positivist form'. Therefore, understanding mixed methods as *only* the combination of qualitative and quantitative methods conflates methodology (the underlying process of knowing, thinking and understanding that guides our questioning and therefore research process) with methods (the techniques used to collect and analyse data). Mixing methods, then, without thinking or acknowledging the underlying theoretical and methodological assumptions of mixing, limits the potential of your strategy for integration – regardless of the individual or cumulative analytical power of the methods mixed.

Quite simply, and as methodological best practice, your methods should be suited to your research question. As I mentioned previously, it was clear that, first, such a topic could not be met through one research method and, second, reducing conceptualising and operationalising processes could not reduce the topic to static, isolatable variables. As such, research questions that require the use of more than one method to answer them will necessarily be broad. Epistemic and ontological tensions in mixed methods research are best dealt with by beginning from an overarching *research problem* manifested in multifaceted research questions that lend themselves to the use of different methods – not just practically but also philosophically.

However, this does not mean you should abandon your sport and exercise science program in order to enrol in philosophy departments before you can undertake your research project. Indeed, Tashakkori and Teddlie are right to be skeptical of the filibustering of philosophers. Rather than avoid the issue, those considering mixed methods research should seriously question what the goal of their research is and how a mixed methods design might produce innovative and important findings.

For example, CrossFit has emerged in recent years as a highly popular physical culture. If I was interested in researching CrossFit's growing popularity and the socio-cultural aspects of the culture, it would seem logical to address several different elements through several different methods, thus creating a mixed methods study. Intuitively, a study of CrossFit could incorporate such things as assessing the physiological impacts of CrossFit training through an experimental design; analysing the commodification of CrossFit through analyses of advertising and production of CrossFit World Championships and developing an understanding of the values, beliefs and behaviours of CrossFit practitioners through ethnographic methods.

The consideration of such a vast array of research methods highlights several competing epistemologies. Yet, in order to develop a holistic understanding of CrossFit, one must take seriously the methodological assumptions and consider the connections between the methods and the research problem in order to avoid merely (re)producing a study of perceived benefits versus 'real' physiological effects. The use of several complimentary research questions better allows the researcher to maintain fidelity to the epistemological and ontological assumptions on which each individual method is based and developed, without simply 'fitting in', at the descriptive level, an extra method or two, in the pursuit of answers.

In my case, the nature of my topic (the relationship between runners and their shoes) really forced me to consider the influence of science on the meaning and experience of being a physically active person, and, therefore, appropriate methods for investigating the relationship between to the two. As such, I was aiming directly at what the founding philosopher of phenomenology, Edmund Husserl, described as the 'crisis of meaning': the gap between the explanatory power of scientific casual accounts and the experience of being human. The overarching problem for my particular project was: How do technology and science influence agency? Substantively, I asked: How do running shoes shape the experience of running? Answering these questions necessitated understanding how shoes were presented to, purchased and used by runners and theorising how technology and science might manifest in these acts.

Ultimately, methodologists' hair splitting over what counts as mixed methods research represents an ideological argument more than an account of best research practices. This is something that is perhaps best articulated by sociologist Howard Becker, who quipped, 'methodology is too important to be left to methodologists' (Becker, 1970, p. 3). That said, most proponents of mixed methods research accept that mixed methods research represents a holistic approach to designing research, which integrates and connects various research methods. Method A plus method B does not equal mixed methods research, regardless of the paradigmatic, academic and historical background of each individual method. Instead, mixed methods research involves the explicit and interconnected use of more than one method in order to answer an overarching research problem. The divide between qualitative and quantitative paradigms is not insurmountable, although it does require serious *methodological* consideration particularly if you are undertaking mixed methods research. Therefore, this chapter takes the same view as Larry Grossberg, who argued: 'I believe that one can and should use any and every kind of empirical method, whatever seems useful to the particular project' (Wright, 2001, p. 145). As such, it is devoted to illustrating how one particular study developed through the inter-connected use of more than one method.

RUNNING BEFORE I COULD WALK: SETTING UP THE STUDY

Following my experience in the running shoe store, I began reviewing both academic and popular literature on running and running shoes in order to better understand my topic. In doing so, I hoped to solidify a research question. I immediately found a meta-analysis by Richards, Magin, and Callister (2009), which found no evidence to suggest that the prescription of running shoes, based on foot type and gait, had any positive biomechanical effect on running. The uncertainty within the positivist paradigm concerning the biomechanical worth of shoe technology, as compared with lay or commonsense knowledge, presented an interesting sociological problem for me to investigate. However, I became dissatisfied with my original plan and decided a mixed methods approach drawing from both quantitative and qualitative methods would enable me to do little more than explore the disconnect between the need for good shoes and their 'actual' impact. Furthermore, I was (and still am) skeptical of the ability of complex theoretical ideas regarding human agency, phenomenology and meaning-making practices to be articulated in a meaningful way through statistical analysis. Therefore, I decided to critically analyse running shoes and running technologies from a sociological perspective by focusing on the socio-cultural dimension, and impacts, of running shoe technology rather than on the impact of running shoes on gait or injury rates.

Such an analysis did not lend itself easily to any one method. As I read more about methods, theory and technology, I realised that designing a study to produce a critical, theoretically generative and empirically grounded analysis of the complex relationship between technology and agency was not a simple task. I sought to bring complementary methods to bear on the subject, not to bolster the findings of each method *per se*, but to illuminate discrete, yet connected, aspects of technology, agency and running. It became clear to me that mixing qualitative methods was the way forward.

With research questions in mind and some ideas about what data would be required in order to produce an answer to my questions, I proceeded to map out a research design that would enable me to better understand and connect idealised running subjectivities with the phenomenological impact of running shoes.

Given that the idea for this project germinated in a trip to purchase a pair of running shoes, ethnography was the research method that made intuitive sense to me. But logistical constraints meant that I was unable to undertake what Taylor (2002) might call 'conventional ethnography' involving 'direct and sustained contact with human agents within the context of their daily lives' (O'Reilly, 2005, p. 3). Therefore, I decided that my desire to produce empirically grounded research that connected my highly personalised experiences with broader social structures would be best met through autoethnography (see Chapter 9). The appeal of an autoethnography, besides its practical suitability, was rooted in its ability to allow critical questioning of running's 'master narrative', which Alexander (2008, p. 92) describes as 'the dominant, hegemonic, way of seeing or thinking the world is or should be the narrative that often guides and undergirds social, cultural, and political mandates'. My anecdotal experiences had instilled in me a desire to evocatively articulate my experiences and understandings rather than produce dry explanations, which cemented autoethnography as the methodological foundation for my research.

If autoethnography made intuitive, as well as practical, sense as a method for exploring what happened when purchasing shoes, then the study of advertising was a natural corollary. Subcultural media were selected as a source of data to explore the discourses and presentation of running shoes and running shoe technology – the reason is that subcultural media represent an important facet of the authentication of popular cultural practice (Wheaton & Beal, 2003). Furthermore, subcultural media are an important marketing tool and, as such, are vital in understanding how running shoes are presented to runners. Therefore, media discourse analysis appealed because it allowed me to inductively identify dominant themes regarding the advertising and use of running shoes as a way to understand the discursive construction of idealised running subjectivities by studying media as both a key reader and generator of running discourse.

When piecing together the mixed methods jigsaw, I found that, for better or worse, there was a large hole in the middle of my design. My research goal was not to create an 'externally valid' study with generalisable results but to gain insight into the role and impact of technology on human agency generally, through a specific study of running shoes. In eschewing positivistic values, I had to ensure that my research captured and expressed some aspect of an intersubjective reality, which Richardson (1999) and other qualitative researchers conceptualise as verisimilitude. The highly personalised impetus for the project and the research design, as it was, provoked further reflection because I felt there was little allowance for the creation of any intersubjective understanding of the relationship between technology and agency in running. Moreover, autoethnography is often criticised for being a reductive and overly subjective method, (ab)used by self-indulgent scholars. Therefore, I decided to supplement my autoethnography with 'traditional' ethnographic methods. The project was, thus, underpinned by ethnographic sensitivities and I drew on a range of methods, including observation, participant-observation and 'ethnographic conversations' (Spradley, 1979) with runners.

Interviews, informal and formal, were used to guide, explain and interpret subcultural media, events and behaviours witnessed during observations. The semi-structured format employed provided the freedom for participants to articulate issues and experiences they deemed important while allowing me to explore interesting and profitable points further, and ensures data are comparable between interviews. Moreover, when conducting ethnographic or autoethnographic fieldwork, it is not always feasible to explicitly discuss the purpose of your research with others. For this reason, I wanted to openly discuss my readings and interpretations of data collected in the field with other runners; thus, interviewing runners became an integral part of the research design.

UP AND RUNNING: GETTING, AND DEALING WITH, DATA

Once I received approval from the University's research ethics board, I began my data collection with excitement. My enthusiasm quickly hit a roadblock. There were only two specialist running stores in town. Conducting fieldwork that would enable me to understand how running shoe technology is negotiated and consumed in running shoe stores would be exceedingly difficult if I continually frequented the same small stores (one of which I recently purchased shoes from), staffed by the same people. It was quite obvious that the owners/staff would begin to wonder what this guy was doing hanging around, not buying anything, pretty quickly. Luckily, London, replete with hundreds of specialty running stores as well as running shoe manufacturers' 'flagship' stores and millions of consumers, was not far away.

Data were collected across a range of stores selling running shoes, which included branded retail outlets, as well as specialist running shops in the English Midlands and London. As such, logic and convenience played a role in sampling. Moreover, I chose running shoe stores because they provide the key empirical context in which runners first come into contact with their running shoes and where they are first exposed to the various technologies that will, literally, shape their bodies. Being in the stores allowed me to experience, first hand, the production of bodily knowledge (through gait analysis) and application of this knowledge (through shoe prescription) and the way this discursively constructs running and promotes certain idealised running practices.

When I was in the stores, I kept field notes quite overtly. My notes included observed events, and notes on such things as the layout of stores and the presentation of shoes. They also included notes from the ethnographic conversations I had with runners and running shoe store staff. To ensure I accurately remembered as much from the conversation as possible, I would record information as soon as reasonably, and politely, possible. This did raise some ethical concerns for me in regards to disclosure and informed consent. I was concerned that disclosure of my research intent might not be appropriate as it could influence the actions, decisions, and behaviours of those I had encountered, thus 'corrupting' data. I never attempted to deceive the people I met in stores and, given that auto-ethnography positions the researcher as the central object of study, I felt comfortable that non-disclosure did not disempower those I interacted with. Moreover, to protect privacy, I presented my analysis as a single monologue.

Analysis was based on personal narrative, which incorporated description, interpretation and explanation. My narrative was constructed through my fieldwork within stores as well as the guided theoretical discussions with runners. That said, I attempted to produce a personalised text about my lived experience of running shoes as presented through running stores by drawing on primary data and my reflection on these experiences. Interpretation required ascertaining the way store layout, marketing and presentation, along with the goals and intentions of sales staff, influenced the presentation of running shoes, the way shoes are explained to runners by staff and forging links between all this to the practice of running. The explanation of these interrelated processes, however, required uncovering the wider implications of personal experience, underpinned by the conceptualisation of social space and techno-scientific discourses.

Advertisements for running shoes provided the data for the media analysis and were collected from two print sources, websites and viral campaigns. My analysis drew on print and internet advertising as an area in which various discourses are mobilised in the service of political agendas to highlight the binaries and fetishisation of technology within running. The goal was to understand what those agendas were, not to produce an all-encompassing representation of all possible discourses. The key print sources, *Runner's World* and *Running Fitness*, were selected on the basis of being the preeminent subcultural texts in terms of volume of readership and geographical distribution in the United Kingdom. I focused on advertisements that presented running shoes as the key product being advertised. Beyond this, my sampling procedure was largely convenience based. Print sources provided the bulk of the sample ($n = 86$), which were composed of advertisements by specific running brands ($n = 75$), running stores advertising multiple shoes ($n = 7$), running shoe buyers' guide supplements ($n = 4$) and web-based sources ($n = 7$). My approach to analysis was heavily influenced by media and communication theories and continued to evolve as my exposure to theory grew, as did the number of advertisements.

Each advertisement was analysed through a close-textual reading (Derrida, 1976) in order to identify dominant themes and the presentation of binaries within advertisements. An ongoing comparative method of textual analysis, involving open and axial coding, was used to divide messages into three main binaries, which quickly became apparent early in the analysis: high technology versus low technology; animal/natural versus human/man made and individual versus group. The development and investigation of each binary was guided by Derridean deconstruction, poststructural interpretations of knowledge claims and critical media theory.

Of particular import was Stuart Hall's (2001) highly influential essay *Encoding/Decoding*, where he outlines connected, but discrete, moments in mass-communication processes in order to draw attention to the difference between semiotic codes imbued in production and the interpretation and evaluation of those codes when texts are read. Hall (2001) refers to these processes as the moments of encoding and decoding, respectively. The moments of encoding and decoding are somewhat linked in the communicative process, but they are also determinate. Consequently, texts are subject to interpretation by audiences – what Fish (1980) has called 'interpretive communities'. Therefore, the message is not conferred through the text itself but rather through the execution of interpretive strategies and the structural maintenance of 'preferred' readings (Hall, 2001). I appreciated that the advertisements I was decoding were polysemic, that is open to many different decodings and subject to interpretation. As such, my decoding was subjective and may have overlooked other binary positions, especially since audience decodings are heterogeneous. Nevertheless, there were dominant meanings and readings of advertisements.

My analysis of running shoe advertisements enabled me to understand the dominant understandings of running practices I was experiencing concomitantly in the stores. I became more and more aware, however, of the need to discuss my readings and understandings with members of the running interpretive community. I found that so much of the process of autoethnography and discourse analysis was dominated by my own background and interpretation that I was concerned that the product of my research would be little more than polemics based on my selective use of corroborating sources. My experiences did not occur in a social, theoretical or methodological vacuum. Therefore, semi-structured interviews became more important in the research process in order to help craft my autoethnography and maximise the verisimilitude of the representation and understanding the meaning making practices of interpretive running communities. As a result, omitting other runners from this project would be illogical and methodologically suspect.

I used 'convenience and criterion purposive sampling' (Miles & Huberman, 1994) to select participants for semi-structured interviews. I wanted runners from a variety of backgrounds and with different motivations, goals for, and experiences of running. I did two 'pilot' interviews to refine my questions, as well as to gain some practice of interviewing before selecting five subjects for formal semi-structured interviews. I selected the participants on the basis of particular characteristics and ability to provide particular insights, as well as unveil individuals' understandings of running shoe technology, in order to gain a variety of perspectives, social backgrounds and running experiences. All lived in England, but they came from various parts of the country and, indeed, world; their running experiences and commitment ranged from someone who jogged for fitness, to someone who had completed over

25 marathons (and counting!), a researcher designing running shoes and a desert ultramarathon runner.

All participants were interviewed at least twice. Interviews were conducted in a range of settings, mostly in pubs and coffee shops. Initial interviews were semi-structured, with approximately 20 questions, with particular emphasis on their experiences using and purchasing running shoes. My questions were constructed in relation to concepts gleaned from the theoretical influences and with reference to my own experiences in running shoe stores. Interviews ranged in length from 50 minutes to 3.5 hours. I used a digital voice recorder during all interviews, made notes during and after interviews, and transcribed the recordings within 24 hours. In this respect, data analysis began as soon as data collection commenced. Veracity of interview data was checked further through transcripts being supplied to participants so that they could identify inaccuracies, misinterpretations or clarify their views; two participants made minor changes to transcripts as a result. The small sample size allowed for in-depth exploration of the lived experiences of runners and their shoes; the depth and richness of the data gained offsets any concerns I might have had with the sample size.

As one might appreciate, organising oneself to get into running stores or pick up the latest *Runner's World* is quite an easy logistical task. Getting someone else to meet you somewhere conducive to conducting interviews is a little more difficult and frustrating. For that reason, interviews did not start until later in the data collection process. This proved to be a blessing in disguise. As concerns rose regarding the highly personal and selective readings of technology and running, I began formally interviewing people about their experiences. Rather than finding more people to interview, I went back to the people I had already interviewed and began to set up secondary and tertiary interviews. These sessions moved away from formally semi-structured interviews and developed into 'guided theoretical dialogues' (Stebbins, 2001), where we explored, more generally, the impact of technology on human behaviour and freedom in late capitalist societies and more specifically, my theoretical readings of how this was reflected in their running practices. This approach required me to lay bare my interpretations of what I was experiencing in running stores, seeing in running advertisements and the themes emerging from initial interviews. Such a process is tricky and challenges you to produce coherent and succinct explanations of often complex theoretical ideas you are only just getting to grips with yourself. Ultimately, I found it a rewarding process as it allowed participants to review, confirm or clarify their narratives incorporated into this project, and also engage with, and explicitly (re)shape, my theoretical positioning and interpretation of data. This strategy really helped give some substance to, and confidence in, my conceptual framework, as well as guided my exploration of theory as used to explain adequately what was happening in the running world. As such, interpretations and understandings were challenged, reinforced, developed and ultimately guided by participants.

As a result of the research process, it became evident to me that technology, as presented through running shoes, is not only the practical application of theoretical knowledge but also, and perhaps more importantly, a particular way of understanding and valuing running and the life world more generally. Running shoe stores and subcultural media both provide important cultural 'touch points' for runners; in so doing, they are important aspects of discursive formation that form the techno-scientific backdrop for running. In this sense, running shoes, as prescribed in running shoe stores, position runners and running as a technical means based procedure, rather than as ends in their own right, with their own intrinsic value. In effect, the presentation and consumption of running shoes creates running practices that attempt to make what is qualitative quantitative and marginalises the meaningful in pursuit of the measurable. More simply, idealised running subjectivities are less about enjoyment, being outside, thrownness (Heidegger, 1962) or flow (Csíkszentmihályi, 1996) than they are about miles covered, calories burned and heart rate zones.

FINAL STEPS: PROMISES, PITFALLS AND FUTURE DIRECTIONS IN MIXED METHODS

Autoethnography began as a way for me to show, rather than tell, the sociological, phenomenological, existential and ontological impact of technology, in the form of running shoes. Nevertheless, it became clear to me that this method alone would not produce a useful understanding of this complex issue, which led me to use a mixed methods design. That said, it is important to note that my use of mixed methods was designed to analyse the various components of this process rather than simply bolster perceived weaknesses in autoethnography. What I present in this chapter is not the single best, or even the only, appropriate use of mixed methods. Indeed, I am not telling you what you should, or should not, be doing when deploying mixed methods or trying to covert you to my particular beliefs about how research should be done or what counts as mixed methods research. Mixed methods made particular sense to me in the context of this particular research project; therefore, I have tried to outline the events that led to my questioning of the way techno-science in both shoes and the prescription process impacts the way we run beyond questions of biomechanical efficiency and the methods I used to try and produce answers to those questions.

Throughout this chapter, I have made much of the practical and logistical issues that shaped the research process. This is something one should be aware of if interested in undertaking a mixed methods project. As the other chapters in this volume articulate clearly, media methods, autoethnography and interviews produce voluminous amounts of data for analysis. The amount of data is, naturally, multiplied when using a mixed methods design. An oft-cited problematic related to mixed methods research is, thus, the contradictory data arising from each method. Contradiction is more likely to be problematic when seeking to triangulate data or methods. There is no one-size-fits-all solution here. Rather than viewing contradiction simply as a 'problem', I think contradictory data highlights an as yet unappreciated complexity to your topic (assuming there are no inherent problems with the design or application of each method) and, as such, present profitable avenues (i.e. theoretical and substantive discovery) for further research. Indeed, for me and this project, I realised that agency and structure are seldom simple propositions – one is rarely totally free to act or exclusively determined by social structures. As such, contradiction highlighted the need for a nuanced understanding of the topic, which led me to guided theoretical discussions as an additional component of the research project. As such, making sense of the immense volume of data proved more difficult than any contradiction therein.

Interestingly, the growth in volume of data in mixed methods designs seems to be exponential rather than linear because not only must the data be connected with the research question but also the various themes in the data must be connected with each other. It was this process that led me to incorporate interviews and guided theoretical discussions into the project in an attempt to better explain these relationships. Each method deployed in this project produced hundreds of pages of notes; connecting the themes and data from each method produced mind maps and diagrams, which resulted in my friends and colleagues describing my workspace as resembling Russell Crowe's shed in the film *A Beautiful Mind*. Do not let this deter you from mixed methods research, however, but do ensure that you are prepared for the amount of data this approach will generate. Thus, you must seriously ask yourself if you have the time necessary to complete not only multiple stages of data collection but also data analysis.

Moreover, the amount of data produced also raises issues should you wish to publish your research. For the sake of meeting word limits when seeking to publish this particular project, I was required to omit the media analysis. This was not an easy decision. However, I felt that the auto-ethnography and guided theoretical dialogues presented the most interesting data, while the media analysis did not produce the same kind of theoretical insight. This is not to say that the media analysis was neither an enlightening nor important part of the research, but rather was not an essential part of the write-up.

The time-consuming nature of mixed methods research, coupled with the need for various types of methodological expertise, means that such research is often conducted as interdisciplinary projects involving more than one researcher. In effect, interdisciplinary research is mixed methods research undertaken by more than one researcher. Such an approach is often touted as something of a necessity for future sport and physical cultural research, especially for qualitative researchers positioned in political and economic climates that demand quantitative measures of research productivity and measure research outputs in terms of acquired funding. Without wishing to be too disparaging of interdisciplinary initiatives, I contend that interdisciplinary research is predicated on simply bringing different methods to bear on the same substantive issue. Interdisciplinary research would do well to learn from mixed methodology, where various methods are explicitly connected and inform one another. This, I hope, is the underlying message this chapter presents. The beauty of mixed methods is that it does allow the various methods to complement one another, to compensate for inherent weaknesses evident in all methods.

However, mixed methods entails more than each method cumulatively reinforcing research findings; such an approach sells mixed methods short and presents a problematic and naïve understanding of both methodology and the ideological and political climate in which we conduct our research. Instead mixed methods research is a reciprocal and recursive approach where the data combined produces a holistic understanding of your topic by seeking to capture the various components of your research problem, not simply corroborating, reconceptualising or operationalising various measurements. As such, the use of mixed methods allows the researcher to produce a coherent research whole that better represents, and, therefore, furthers understanding of, the complex political, social, cultural and historical trajectories, values and bodies at play in SPCs.

FIVE KEY READINGS

1. Giddings, L. (2006). Mixed-methods research: Positivism dressed in drag? *Journal of Research in Nursing, 11*(13), 195–203.
A self-identified mixed methodologist presents a succinct and jargon-free text that outlines the political and ideological fault lines evident in the methodology of mixed methods. Championing co-operative and complex research designs to address complex issues in health, this paper will be of special interest to those who approach a mixed methods design with critical and interpretive methods and theories as cornerstones of their project.

2. Huemer, M. (Ed.) (2002). *Epistemology: Contemporary Readings.* **London: Routledge.**
Producing mixed methods research requires serious consideration of paradigmatic and epistemological tensions within the research design and the philosophical foundation of the individual methods deployed. This edited collection draws on the musings of influential philosophers, both classic and contemporary, and their analyses provide an excellent place to start the careful and considerate reflection on all things epistemic and ontological that putting together a mixed methodology demands.

3. Roethlisberger, F. J., & Dickson, W. J. (1939). *Management and the worker: An account of a research program conducted by the Western electric company, Hawthorne Works, Chicago.* **Cambridge: Harvard University Press.**
The now infamous study from which the notion of the Hawthorne Effect (reactivity based on knowledge of being studied) is named. Field experiments, observational studies and interviews were used in this seminal mixed methods study.

4. Somekh, B., & Lewin, C. (2010) *Theory and Methods in Social Research* **(2nd ed.) Thousand Oaks, CA: Sage.**
This edited collection provides an introduction to a range of qualitative and quantitative research techniques as well as illustrations of how they might be combined in and through mixed methods research. Expansive reading lists make this a good place to find information on a range of methods that can be deployed in mixed methods studies of SPC.

5. Tashakkori, A., & Teddlie, C. (2010). *Handbook of mixed methods in social and behavioral research* **(2nd ed.). Thousand Oaks, CA: Sage.**
This *handbook* focuses primarily on mixed methods research as composed of qualitative and quantitative methods, but remains primary reading for

researchers serious about designing mixed methods or 'multi-methods' research. Examples ranging from social to health sciences highlight the empirical, methodological, epistemological and theoretical tensions in mixed methods research alongside prosaic advice on design, logistical and procedural issues.

REFERENCES

Alexander, B. K. (2008). Performance ethnography: The re-enacting and inciting of culture. In N. K. Denzin & Y. S. Lincoln (Eds.), *The SAGE handbook of qualitative research* (3rd ed., pp. 75–118). Thousand Oaks, CA: Sage.

Becker, H. S. (1970). *Sociological work: Method and substance.* Chicago, IL: Aldine Publishing Company.

Besculides, M., Zaveri, H., Farris, R., & Will, J. (2006). Identifying best practices for WISEWOMAN programs using a mixed-methods evaluation. *Preventing Chronic Disease: Public Health Research, Practice, and Policy, 3*(1), 1–9.

Collins, M. (2011). The politics of the environment, and noisy sports: Two totally different outcomes in the Lake District National Park for powerboating and off-road motoring. *Leisure Studies, 30*(4), 423–452.

Csíkszentmihályi, M. (1996). *Creativity: Flow and the psychology of discovery and invention.* New York: Harper Perennial.

Denzin, N. K. (1978). The logic of naturalistic inquiry. In N. K. Denzin (Ed.), *Sociological methods: A sourcebook* (pp. 166–182). New York: McGraw-Hill.

Derrida, J. (1976). *Of grammatology.* Baltimore, MD: Johns Hopkins University Press.

Fish, S. E. (1980). *Is there a text in this class? The authority of interpretive communities.* Cambridge: Harvard University Press.

Fortier, M., Hogg, W., O'Sullivan, T., Blanchard, C., Reid, R., Sigal, R., ... Beaulac, J. (2007). The physical activity counselling (PAC) randomized controlled trial: Rationale, methods, and interventions. *Applied Physiology, Nutrition and Metabolism, 32,* 1170–1185.

Geertz, C. (1973). *The Interpretation of cultures.* New York: Basics Books.

Gmelch, G. (1978). Magic in professional baseball. In G. P. Stone (Ed.), *Games, sports, and power,* (pp. 128–137). New Brunswick, NJ: Dutton.

Green, J., Kreider, H., & Mayer, E. (2011). Combining qualitative and quantitative methods in social inquiry. In B. Somekh & C. Lewin (Eds.), *Theory and methods in social research* (2nd ed., pp. 259–267). Thousand Oaks, CA: Sage.

Hall, S. (2001). Encoding/Decoding. In M. G. Durham & D. Kellner (Eds.), *Media and cultural studies: Key works* (pp. 166–176). Oxford: Blackwell.

Heidegger, M. (1962). *Being in time.* Oxford: Blackwell.

John, A., & Jackson, S. (2010). Call me loyal: Globalization, corporate nationalism and the America's cup. *International Review for the Sociology of Sport, 46*(4), 339–417.

Lynd, R. S., & Lynd, H. M. (1927). *Middletown.* New York: Harcourt.

Miles, M., & Huberman, A. (1994). *Qualitative data analysis* (2nd ed.). London: Sage.

O'Reilly, K. (2005). *Key concepts in ethnography.* London: Sage.

Polsky, N. (1967). *Hustlers, beats, and others.* Chicago, IL: Aldine Publishing Company.

Richards, C. E., Magin, P. J., & Callister, R. (2009). Is your prescription of distance running shoes evidence-based? *British Journal of Sports Medicine, 43*(3), 159–162.

Richardson, L. (1999). Feathers in our CAP. *Journal of Contemporary Ethnography, 28,* 660–668.

Roethlisberger, F. J., & Dickson, W. J. (1939). *Management and the worker: An account of a research program conducted by the Western electric company, Hawthorne Works, Chicago.* Cambridge: Harvard University Press.

Scott, M. B. (1968). *The racing game.* Chicago, IL: Aldine Publishing Company.

Spradley, J. P. (1979). *The ethnographic interview.* New York: Holt, Rinehart and Winston.

Stebbins, R. (2001). *Exploratory research in the social sciences.* London: Sage.

Stranger, M. (2011). *Surfing life: Surface, substructure and the commodification of the sublime.* Surrey, UK: Ashgate.

Taylor, S. (2002). *Ethnographic research: A reader.* London: Sage.

Teddlie, C., & Tashakkori, A. (2010). Major issues and controversies in the use of mixed methods in the social and behavioral sciences. In A. Tashakkori & C. Teddlie (Eds.), *Handbook of mixed methods in social and behavioral research* (2nd ed., pp. 3–50). Thousand Oaks, CA: Sage.

Tjomsland, H. (2010). Sustaining comprehensive physical activity practice in elementary school: A case study applying mixed methods. *Teachers and Teaching: Theory and Practice, 16*(1), 73–95.

Wheaton, B., & Beal, B. (2003). Keeping it real: Subcultural media and the discourses of authenticity in alternative sport. *International Review for the Sociology of Sport, 38*(2), 155–176.

Woodward, K. (2009). Hanging out and hanging about: Insider/outsider research in the sport of boxing. *Ethnography, Physical Culture, 9*(4), 536–560.

Wright, K. H. (2001). "What's going on?" Larry Grossberg on the status quo of cultural studies: An interview. *Cultural Values, 5*(2), 133–162.

CHAPTER 11

TRUTH OR DARE: EXAMINING THE PERILS, PAINS AND PITFALLS OF INVESTIGATIVE METHODOLOGIES IN THE SOCIOLOGY OF SPORT

John Sugden

ABSTRACT

Purpose – *Good investigative sociology and high-quality investigative journalism are not just the same but they are close relatives. For both professions, getting under the surface soil of social life, digging deeply into and making coherent sense of the social experience of others, and translating those findings and interpretations into a universal language for widespread consumption are hugely challenging tasks. Understanding the difference and similarities regarding how sociologists and investigative journalists go about this task raises fundamental philosophical, epistemological, ethical, methodological, theoretical and practical concerns, the outline considerations of which are all featured in this chapter.*

Design/methodology/approach – *Drawing upon more than three decades of investigative research experience in the field and the original and the innovative personal scholarship that this has yielded, the chapter offers*

Qualitative Research on Sport and Physical Culture
Research in the Sociology of Sport, Volume 6, 233–252
Copyright © 2012 by Emerald Group Publishing Limited
All rights of reproduction in any form reserved
ISSN: 1476-2854/doi:10.1108/S1476-2854(2012)0000006014

students a map reader's guide of how to navigate a way through the complex, challenging and sometimes hazardous labyrinth of investigative qualitative research.

Originality/value – *In addition to offering a 'how to' primer for thinking about and doing investigative-qualitative sociology, the chapter also offers advice on how to survive the experience and authoritatively tell the tale well to the widest possible audiences.*

Keywords: Investigative sociology; epistemology; research ethics; risk assessment; intellectual craftsmanship

INTRODUCTION

In a leading article for the British Sociological Association (BSA) Newsletter, Ivor Gaber, freelance journalist and Emeritus Professor of Broadcast Journalism (Gaber, 2003) at Goldsmiths College, University of London, suggested that sociologists might improve their skills of interpretation and communication by developing closer relations with journalism, particularly investigative journalism. In this chapter, I will be reflecting upon Gaber's position and exemplifying issues that have emerged through my own fieldwork: researching, among other things, transnational boxing subcultures (Sugden, 1996), the governing body of world football, FIFA (Sugden & Tomlinson, 1998, 1999, 2003), and the 'black economy' that has grown in the shadows of the same game (Sugden, 2002). Much of this output inhabits a grey area between investigative journalism and investigative sociology. Trying to make sense of the differences and similarities between the two professions raises a series of epistemological, ethical and methodological issues: beginning with the most problematic question of all – what is truth?[1]

SEARCHING FOR THE TRUTH

According to Hugo De Burgh, investigative journalists are usually driven people whose mission it is to probe into, and uncover, corruption, malpractice and abuse of power usually in corporate, government and/or criminal settings:

> Investigative journalists attempt to get at the truth where the truth is obscure because it suits others that it be so; they choose their topics from a sense of right and wrong which we can only call a moral sense, but in the manner of their research they attempt to be

dispassionately evidential. They are doing more than disagreeing with how society runs; they are pointing out that it is failing by its own standards. They expose, but they expose in the public interest, which they define. Their efforts, if successful, alert us to failures in the system and lead to politicians, lawyers and policemen taking action. (2000, p. 23)

In this formulation, one is immediately struck by the unproblematic notion of truth that fires the investigative journalist's imagination. For them, the truth is a taken-for-granted fact that is unquestionably out there: the problem is finding truth and revealing it. Some sociologists, on the other hand, in a post-postmodern moment, are so hung up on the philosophical questions of what is truth and who can legitimately seek it; we are sometimes reluctant to take to the field in the first place. Of course, there is nothing new in sociological and philosophical debates about the notion of truth and objectivity. Indeed, it could be argued that searching for the answer to this question has been the cornerstone of philosophy, ancient and modern. However, while the philosopher's muse about truth can be the central to their discipline, an inability to get beyond it is a major impediment to the business of social science, which is an essentially empirical (not empiricist) enterprise.

The pursuit of empirical truth has not been helped by the postmodernist turn that impacted upon sociology and cultural studies in the 1980s and 1990s. Within a postmodernist cultural studies, the empirically based quest to delineate and theorise the lived nature of social relations has been overwhelmed by an obsession with deconstructing 'texts' *and* 'discourses', at the expense of trying to make sense of the social worlds of those who constructed them (Lash, 1999). Other critiques of positivism (Ward, 1997) privilege a standpoint epistemology which holds that only those who embody and live through the identities and experiences under scrutiny can have sufficient empathetic understanding to construct adequate interpretations – for instance, 'that women's subjugation puts them in a privileged position to produce true knowledge of women's subjugation' (Wacquant, 1993, p. 497). To follow this principle effectively means that only women can study women, only black people black people and, presumably, only football hooligans football hooligans and so on. Surely, however, to adopt such an epistemological and ontological position takes away the interpretative role of the sociologist. It makes of sociological readings of life a series of generated accounts in which, say, experiential narratives are not necessarily related to the wider social picture.

There will always be problems with any relativist position that privileges the assumed authenticity of any single voice.[2] Detached critique and evidence-informed scepticism are necessary for the defence of an associational realism upon which the metalanguage of the critical social science community is based. Willis, for instance, in his seminal ethnographic work, *Learning to Labour* (1977), never left the voices of his subjects to speak merely for themselves. His ethnography of the lads is mediated by his interpretative conceptualising intervention, and then – separately – densely theorised in the metalanguage of social science, and so avoids falling into any reductionist relativism or romantic celebration of the voices of the less powerful. I hesitate to introduce the term 'objectivity' into this debate as it has been out of sociological fashion for a number of years. While agreeing with the idea that it is impossible to be fully objective – that is, to arrest and lock away our own ideological baggage and fully blinker the ensuing gaze – that when doing sociological research, particularly when it involves intimate social contact with segments of social life that we do not naturally inhabit, I continue to believe that attempting to be as objective as one can possibly be in the circumstances one finds oneself should be a guiding aspiration when in the field. Yes, come clean to yourself about your position as researcher, but do not allow this to dominate your capacity for honest and dis-passionate interpretation.

SOCIOLOGICAL IMPRESSIONISM

Investigative sociologists should have a commitment to the objective, rigorous and systematic quest for truth. This, however, can never be the philosophical or absolute truth that Ward seems to be talking about or the uncritical notion of truth which works for journalists. Rather it is a sociological truth. Clegg (2000) argues that whereas the former asks what is truth (a question that Foucault believed unanswerable), sociological truth is 'what passes for truth' (p. 141) – in other words, what people believe to be true in the context of the social worlds within which they abide. Given this formulation, and given that there are multiple vantage points, there are multiple *truths*. In the context of particular social hierarchies and networks of power, it is the task of the researcher to identify, gain access to and share as many of these vantage points as possible. On this basis, it is possible to construct an overall interpretation that may not be true to any single vantage point, but which, by taking account of them all, including that of the researcher, is the most honest representation of a given milieu's shared truth about itself at a given point in history. This approach can be explained through an artistic metaphor:

> To clarify this, think of the difference between a photograph and an impressionist painter's canvas. The photograph captures a moment of reality (or truth) that is

immediately transient, and dependent on prevailing and instantly passing conditions of light, shade, expression and so forth. And remember, just like respondents in interviews, the camera can lie. The impressionist painting, on the other hand, is constructed over time and incorporates the various dimensions of the artist's gaze and what is known about the places and people that are painted. It also leaves room for interpretation by those who view the work in the gallery. Thus, what is produced is not reality per se, but an informed *impression* of that reality. The artist then offers the painting for public appraisal, acclaim or ridicule, implicitly challenging other artists to depict the chosen scene differently. In this way we regard ourselves as rigorous social scientists and as *social impressionists.* (Sugden & Tomlinson, 2002, p. 18)

McDonald makes a further and useful distinction between radical and moralistic epistemological positions stating, 'moralistic social research collapses the boundaries between research and activism' (McDonald, 2002, p. 114). People working in this way not only privilege the voices of the oppressed but manipulate those voices to serve their own activist agendas: 'Little attention is paid to the conventions of sound scholarly habits, which are dismissed anyway as elitist and bogus, as the aim of research is to support the attainment of immediate political goals' (*ibid.*). The radical approach, on the other hand, while likewise having an explicit political agenda, incorporates this as one perspective amongst many and accounts for it as part of multilayered process of getting at the sociological truth:

Underpinning this approach is a view that there is no special virtue in those that lack power and authority, and more than in those who possess them. In particular, there is no reason to believe that the perspective of those placed the bottom of society is more likely to be true than those at the top. (McDonald, 2002, p. 109)

Adopting a left-realist position, McDonald argues the following: by all means let politics set the sociological agenda and encourage others (and ourselves as activists if necessary) to use the yield of sociological enquiry to promote equitable social change. Do not, however, allow this to influence the methods through which we gather and present the evidence and argument.

THE FOURTH ESTATE AND THE INVESTIGATIVE IMPERATIVE IN SOCIOLOGICAL RESEARCH

This brings us to another key question: how do you get at sociological truth if those who inhabit it do not want to give it up? To begin with the term 'investigative sociology' is somewhat tautological inasmuch as sociology is (or should be) by its very nature investigative in its mission to discover,

uncover and make sense of the mysteries and complexities of social life. Be
that as it may, this is not a view remembered or widely shared among many
contemporaries calling themselves sociologists. Thus, investigative sociology
is an important methodological tradition in need of revival because passive
forms of ethnography – that is fieldwork in which the researcher's role is
dictated and constrained by the flow of events presented to him or her as
'natural' – rarely allows for the full impressionist canvas to be filled.
Investigative sociological research is an important dimension of the critical
gaze. It is not a new category (although, it has for some years lain dormant
within the social scientist's methodological repertoire).

In the 1960s and 1970s, Jack Douglas, a sociologist at the University of
California, retrieved this tradition, arguing that any valid critique of what
is really going on must go beyond passive observation and embrace the
investigative. His investigative mission combines a quest for truth with the
recognition that observation is essential: 'Direct observation of things in
their natural state (uncontrolled) is the primary basis of all truth ... this
bedrock facticity of concrete experience and observation pervades our
everyday lives' (Douglas, 1976, p. 12). To get at the truth, direct observation, for Douglas, necessarily goes beyond gazing at the surface. His
'conflict methodological' research strategy is based upon the assumption
that everyday social life has a tendency to be duplicitous: that individuals
and groups construct and present images of who they are and what they do
that can mask underpinning social realities:

> The investigative paradigm is based upon the assumption that profound conflicts of
> interest, values, feelings and actions pervade social life. It is taken for granted that
> many of the people one deals with, perhaps all people to some extent, have good
> reason to hide from others what they are doing and even lie to them. Instead of
> trusting people and expecting trust in return, one suspects others and expects others to
> suspect him. Conflict is the reality of life; suspicion is the guiding principle. (Douglas,
> 1976, p. 55)

Douglas's view of the nature of social life is framed by his experience of
researching relatively microscopic, albeit 'deviant' subcultures. However, his
basic principles can be taken to apply to all walks of life. He does not believe
that all people are fraudulent all of the time, but he does maintain that even
the most trivial areas of social interaction can be distorted through
combinations of misinformation, evasions, outright lies and stage management. He argues that social research must account for this and advocates mixed methodologies that are simultaneously 'cooperative and
investigative' (Douglas, 1976, p. 56) – that is methodologies that take note

of self-generated and freely given legends, but that also subject such 'official histories' to scrutiny from a multitude of vantage points.

Classic subcultural studies by former newspaper reporter, Robert Park, and his contemporaries in the Chicago School in the 1920s and 1930s were, in part, dependent upon the methods of investigative and muck-raking journalism – a tradition that can be traced back to Charles Dickens and beyond (de Burgh, 2000). This style of reformist political and corporate whistle-blowing made an important contribution to public accountability and the protection of democratic process in the nineteenth and early twentieth centuries on both sides of the Atlantic (Kaplan, 1975).

Investigative journalists schooled in this tradition tend to view themselves then as keepers of the public conscience. Mathew Kieran argued that 'journalism can usefully be characterised, in part, as an official Fourth Estate which has the function of pursuing and covering stories that concern the political legal or social interests of the public as citizens … The basic Lockean thought is that citizens must be made aware of the nature, workings, and character of those in government so they are in a position to exercise their will as citizens and judge those to whom power is entrusted on their behalf' (2000, p. 156). While the Washington Post's Watergate investigations that brought about the downfall of US President Richard Nixon in the 1970s is the most outstanding example of this kind of work (Woodwar & Bernstein, 1981), the investigative imperative is not, and should not be, restricted to the confines of formal political parties and related organisations, rather it should pervade all aspects of social life where it is the public's interest to know exactly what is going on.

The aim to penetrate, interpret and, where relevant, make transparent the inner workings of public and private corporate organisations is too important a task to be left to journalists alone. Today, the global media are dominated by fewer and fewer self-interested and self-censoring conglom- erates (Said, 1993). According to John Pilger (1999), investigative journalists are a threatened species. They are being crowded out, to be replaced by automata masquerading as news reporters. With notable exceptions, such as the works of Andrew Jennings in the United Kingdom and Dave Zarin in the United States, investigative journalism has also been pushed further to the margins of mainstream sports reporting. One of the chief reasons for this is the power of sport organisations and their 'PR minders' to freeze out journalists who ask too many *unpleasantly* probing questions, the subtext being, be nice to us or it's 'access denied'. Jennings himself is a well-known victim of such exclusionary tactics. While the advent of rebellious forms of multi-platform e-journalism – and both Jennings and Zirin are pioneers in this field[3] – promises to open new fronts in the battle for transparency and accountability in corporate sport, for the time being it is more important than ever that we give space in our journals to the critical voices of sport academics to be heard alongside those of a dwindling and endangered band of investigative journalists. The freedom of the press is likewise under threat as ideology and 'spin' replace factual news and critical analysis. The more that the independence of the Fourth Estate it is threatened, the more important it is that sociologists, at least occasionally, leave the relative sanctuary of the academy and reinvigorate the investigative tradition. Sociology has indeed made a significant contribution to this Fourth Estate. Some of my own work, particularly that with Alan Tomlinson, on power, politics and corruption within the governing body of world football, FIFA, for instance, is justified and driven by such Lockean principles:

> This book is not an epitaph for the people's game. We have written it because we believe that information is power. Pointing out who is doing what to your game, we believe that we can make a valuable contribution to the growing resistance and reaction against the total commodification of football. (Sugden & Tomlinson, 1999, p. 8)

PROSE NOT POSE

Unlike sociologists, investigative journalists do not usually target the ordinary or mundane aspects of everyday life. Sociologists' interest may include high-level corporate malpractice, but it also may embrace much less spectacular, nonetheless interesting spheres of social life, following social anthropologist Alan Klein's (1993) advice and making the exotic appear ordinary and the ordinary exotic. For instance, the social construction of status, identity and meaning among groups of volunteer charity workers may hold some fascination for certain sociologists and may lend itself to an investigative approach, but it is unlikely to fire the imagination of an investigative reporter. Neither are investigative journalists so much concerned with the broader concerns of social structure and social process that frame and help to account for the kind of corruption and injustice that they choose to expose. In other words, their commentaries lack any theoretical gravity. It would be a brave (and soon to be unemployed) newspaper reporter of even the most respected and highbrow broadsheet that attempted to invoke Bourdieu and Focault in his feature on power and corruption in local government! In this context, in some of my own work I have felt the wrath of sceptical editors and publishers. Once I submitted a book proposal to a publisher in the popular market. The idea for a book on football and the underground economy was warmly embraced apart from the last chapter in which I proposed to flesh out first-level narratives, characterisations and interpretations with broader theoretical issues and social-structural connections. The publisher in question agreed to publish the book (Sugden, 2002), and even offered me a modest advance, so long, that is I omitted the final chapter! Of course, this has as much to do with target audiences as it does with the substance of enquiry and mode of analysis.

This raises another obvious, and in my view, regrettable, distinction between journalists and sociologists. The former are usually much better communicators. Journalists write for the general public, whereas sociologists usually write for more specialist and sociologically sensitised audiences. The latter, however, can be no excuse for the amount of impenetrable jargon that characterises much contemporary sociology. If sociologists are to make a contribution to the preservation and development of democracy, they need to find voices that can be heard and understood. For some, sociology has developed into a kind of *Glass Bead Game* whereby primacy is given to the demonstration of general theoretical sophistication over the empirical analysis of social phenomena. The *Glass Bead Game* is the fictional creation of German novelist and philosopher Herman Hesse who describes it thus:

> The only way to learn the rules of this Games of games is to take the usual prescribed course, which requires many years, and none of the initiates could ever possibly have any interest in making those rules easier to learn. These rules, the sign language and grammar of the Game, constitute a kind of highly developed secret language. (Hesse, 1970, p. 18)

As Orwell argued vigorously, assumed technical sophistication is no excuse for bad English (1994). Orwell's tirade was directed towards political commentaries of his day. Surely, however, of all the academic disciplines, with the possible exception of English itself, sociology – the study of society – should be the most accessible of subjects. That it is not is nothing short of shameful. A view endorsed by C. Wright Mills who, in a searing critique of some of his contemporaries, said:

> To overcome academic prose, you must first overcome academic pose ... To be called a 'mere journalist' makes him feel undignified and shallow. It is this situation, I think, that is often at the bottom of the elaborate vocabulary and involved manner of speaking and writing ... It may be that it is the result of an academic closing of ranks on the part of the mediocre, who understandably wish to exclude those who win the attention of intelligent people, intelligent or otherwise. (1970, p. 240)

Wright Mills was a very widely read scholar who had a supreme command of the classic tradition in nineteenth and twentieth century sociology. But as he demonstrates amply through his own research and writing, there is no good reason why the possession of a highly tuned *sociological imagination* and the capacity to write clearly and succinctly should be mutually exclusive talents. Instead, he used his encyclopaedic knowledge of social theory as a kind of intellectual scaffolding within which to frame and craft his own interpretations and theories: once finished, like a house builder putting a new home on the market, he removed the scaffolding to reveal his distinctive contribution to the body of knowledge.

ETHNOGRAPHY AND ETHICS

Journalism is by no means all virtue. On the contrary, driven by circulation statistics and headline hungry editors, journalists, unlike most (but not all) sociologists, can become over-dependent upon sensationalist expose and juicy stories. The danger here is that too often the journalist is tempted to use sources that are either too narrowly focussed and/or required degrees of anonymity that make verification impossible. It may also encourage a resort to tactics that are not normally associated with the sociologists' method. This would include such things as 'check book journalism', 'faction' (dramatic reconstruction of events that are alleged to have taken place), 'stings' (entrapment operations) and a wide ranging of techniques based on deception. At worst it can lead journalists to fabrication – never let the truth get in the way of a good story!

If ever there were any doubts about this, the phone hacking scandals that engulfed the British press in 2011 (which, in its wake, brought down Rupert Murdoch's *The News of the World* – one of Britain's oldest and best selling Sunday newspapers) wiped such doubts away. Central to the ensuing investigations and cross-party parliamentary hearings was the need to clarify the distinction between stories that were deemed to be in the public interest and those that were merely interesting to the public. While the former gives a far greater moral conviction for reporters to use any number of devious means to go after their stories, the latter does not. The problems associated with the evocation of a public interest clause in doing certain forms of investigative sociological research will be discussed later in this chapter.

Verification and reliability are much more important principles for sociologists who are required to present in full context that lies behind the headlines. We must demonstrate in detail how we gather our data and what sources we have used so that those who come after us can replicate our studies and test our findings and interpretations. Necessarily, however, this must go beyond a reliance on official sources and self-generated biographies/hagiographies and glossy institutional histories: sources that are notoriously unreliable. In order to cover all of the angles – access all of the vantage points that comprise a sociological truth – sometimes it is necessary to resort to, or at least take advantage of, forms of deception. I must confess that more than once while in the field, I have pretended to be other than I am in order to get inside organisations and gangs and to get deep access to insider information that would have otherwise been withheld.

This raises another important set of issues that require some thought and discussion. What, if anything, are or should be the differences in the ethical principles that underpin the regulation of investigative journalists' method compared to those of sociology? This is a very grey area. Sociologists, in the United Kingdom at least, are advised rather than regulated through the BSA's 'Statement of Ethical Practice' (BSA, 2002). This is, to say the least, an ambiguous document that has not been written with the investigative sociologist in mind. The over-riding emphasis is towards the protection of those studied and their empowerment in terms of the way data collected from and about them are interpreted, communicated and disseminated. Take clause 24, for example, which states that 'Clarification should also be given to research participants regarding the degree to which they will be consulted prior to publication. Where possible, participants should be offered feedback on findings' (*ibid.*, p. 6). The spirit of this clause is hard to square with some of the underlying assumptions of investigative sociology outlined previously. If even in relatively mundane spheres of social activity, individuals and groups hold views of themselves that are underpinned by self-interest, it is difficult to imagine how those same individuals and groups could be allowed to influence the researcher's interpretation of findings without undermining the search for sociological truth. This problem is magnified when researching large official groups and organisations (such as, for instance, FIFA or Manchester United) that have PR departments with communications directors (spin doctors), the sole purpose of which is to promote 'squeaky clean' official histories that deflect attention from corruption and malpractice. Likewise, the veracity of our investigations into so-called deviant and/or criminal subcultures is unlikely to be enhanced by ongoing consultations with subjects with regards to the images of their worlds that we are constructing.

There is also the related issue of how a researcher is supposed to go about gathering insider information. Wherever possible, we are advised to be candid with our research hosts about the nature of our research and our role as researchers. Usually access to a research setting is gained via a 'gate-keeper'. In these situations, the BSA reminds us: 'members should adhere to the principle of gaining informed consent directly from the research participants to whom access is required, while at the same time taking account of the gatekeepers' interest' (*ibid.*). This consent, we are told, should be 'regarded, not as a once and for all prior event, but as a process subject to renegotiation over time. In addition, particular care may need to be taken during periods of prolonged fieldwork where it is easy for research participants to forget that they are being studied' (*ibid.*).

Much of my own research experience has led me to take the opposite view. Wherever possible, I have avoided fully covert work. Not only, as the BSA makes clear (*ibid.*, p. 9), is this very problematic ethically, but it is also very risky, especially when working in potentially dangerous settings involving people who are suspicious of those who would study them. I have reached the conclusion that the most productive, and certainly the most secure *modus operandi* for investigative sociology is to let a few key informants know up-front, without going into too much detail, that you are a researcher. Then, as the fieldwork progresses, make it easy for them to forget by fading into the background and becoming part of the furniture. This allows for a greater sense of sociological naturalism to pervade the fieldwork.

Also, I have occasionally found it useful to be less than fully honest, and in some cases dishonest, about my research interests and where the product of my research will be disseminated. When embarking on our FIFA work, for instance, Alan Tomlinson and I told potential gatekeepers that we were social historians, not sociologists, the latter being regarded with some suspicion in the corporate world. The idea of academics producing a social history of some or other institution is far less threatening than the prospect of a potentially revealing and acerbic sociological analysis and critique, which our various FIFA publications tended to be. In addition, in circumstances such as this, it proved to be useful to encourage a belief that the yield of our studies was targeted for a strictly academic clientele. Similarly, for my football-black economy research, my key gatekeeper assumed that the product of my fieldwork would end up gathering dust on a university library shelf. I did little to discourage that view as it helped me with ongoing insider access. That it ended up in paperback and sold thousands of copies on the high street was, as we shall discover, a very unpleasant surprise for my hosts.

FLATTERY AND BETRAYAL

One thing that investigative sociologists and journalists have in common is the resort to interpersonal treachery. In my experience, in order to gain full empathetic access to the world of the other, it is useful to develop a positive rapport with them. To achieve this, it is important to find and focus upon an aspect of their character that you can at least pretend to like. Some of the subjects of my research have been, in my view, pretty reprehensible, but I have almost always discovered in them something that I can relate to. By cutting out the bad and the ugly and homing in on the good, the researcher can develop a lines of communication through which the required inform- ation can flow more freely. This is the stock in trade of most 'fly-on-the-wall' television documentary makers, but it can also be a useful strategy for investigative sociologists. For both the researcher and the researched, however, this is an uncomfortable manipulation of the natural human desire for facilitation and friendship. In the end, because the subjects of investi- gative sociology can be exposed to public scrutiny in ways that either make them look foolish, bad, or both, such intimate research relationships can end with a deep sense of betrayal. I am absolutely certain that key gatekeepers in FIFA and in the football-black market felt betrayed once they read what had been written about them and the networks of which they were guardians. According to Tomlinson, this is something that comes with the turf:

> However much the researcher subscribes to the ethical principles of a research discipline, in the messy world of social research at least, the integrity of the project should be at the forefront of the researcher's consideration. The social researcher, despite and argot of methodological reflexivity behind which moral issues might be veiled, faces the same moral issues as the investigative reporter ... to sense that the subject or respondent has been flattered and betrayed is to sensitively recognise the strengths of oral sources and use them critically. Merely to produce an oral account, or to over-anonymise it, would be a greater betrayal of the very task of interpretation. (1997, p. 262)

THE PUBLIC INTEREST

Using deceit in the service of sociology, however, requires ethical justification that goes beyond 'for the integrity of the project'. Once more, the BSA's guidelines are ambiguous. On the one hand, we are told: 'research relationships should be characterised by trust and integrity ... although sociologists, like other researchers are committed to the advancement of knowledge, that goal does not, of itself, provide and entitlement to override the rights of others' (2002, p. 16). In the same code of practice, we are offered the following 'get-out' clause: 'in some cases, where the public interest dictates otherwise and particularly where power is being abused, obligations of trust and protection may weigh less heavily. Nevertheless, these obligations should be discarded lightly' (*ibid.*, p. 4) – hardly a ringing endorsement of the methods of investigative sociology.

Journalists, who are regulated through a variety of codes of conduct/ practice, are subject to similar ethical considerations. However, there is less ambiguity when it comes to the question of matters deemed to be in the public interest. The public interest as defined by the PCC (Press Complaints Commission) includes 'detecting or exposing crime or serious misdemea- nour; protecting public health and safety; preventing the public from being misled by some statement or action of an individual or organisation' (1997, p. 1). Once, it seems, journalists have established that the focus of their inquiries are 'in the public interest', then, to a large extent, the end – that is publication and exposure – justifies the means.

As Kiernan argues:

> ... one might think at various points investigative journalists, to be effective as such, will have to be immoral ... very often successfully investigating hidden scandals or corruption requires journalists to misrepresent themselves, deceive, lie, intrude into privacy and in extreme cases even break the law, all actions we normally presume are wrong. If investigative journalism were required to be morally good they would be unable to penetrate the murky world they need to investigate and thus would be unable to do their job. It is something like this that thought that underlies the presumption of may journalists that at a certain point ethical considerations are excluded from the sphere of investigative journalism. (2000, p. 158)

Kiernan goes onto argue, however, that immoral actions used in the service of investigative journalism are only justifiable if the moral purpose for doing so is incontrovertible (*ibid.*, 159). When conducting in-depth sociological investigations into the affairs of individuals, groups and organisations that are clearly in the publics' interest to know about, it is my contention that the same flexible approach should be taken. I have argued elsewhere that 'getting one's hands dirty' does not mean that the investigator has become morally corrupt (Sugden & Tomlinson, 1999). As is the case with journalism, however, such strategies should only be deployed as a last resort when they are the only way through which to establish evidence of neglect, corruption and/or criminal practise that has resulted or may result in significant harm to others or undermine the commonwealth.

Without such license, the sociologists' capacity to make meaning contributions to social policy and social change is undermined.

The ethical context for investigative research is a very grey area that, in my experience, is a question of principle and balance that can only be worked out in practice. I have in the past, for instance, turned down the opportunity to misappropriate important documents, even though they might have shed important light on the subject of my inquiry, largely because of the consequences that might befall the person who left them unguarded. In other situations, I have participated in black market activities (for no personal gain) when I judged that this would get me deeper inside the subcultural world that I was investigating without resulting in any substantial harm to others. In this case I believed that the story was worth, in public interest terms, the marginal immorality and the issue for the next section: the risk to others and to me.

RISK ASSESSMENT

There are two dimensions to this issue of risk in fieldwork: risk to the researched and risk to the researcher. In several places, the BSA warns us that we have a duty of care to those who we study, not just while we are in the field, but also after we have left it: 'Members have a responsibility both to safeguard the proper interests of those involved in or affected by their work ... they need to consider the effects of their involvements and the consequences of their work or its misuse for those they study' (BSA, p. 2). No matter how much we would choose to avoid it, almost by definition investigative sociology can run the risk of damaging the quality of life of some of those that we have studied. Gatekeepers can be especially vulnerable because it is they who let us in and often bear the brunt of the blame once we have left and told the company secrets. For the work on FIFA, for instance, Alan Tomlinson and I (remember, posturing as historians) benefited considerably from the co-operation of the organisation's director of communications who was not just a key informant but also a very important gatekeeper. Not long after our second book on the subject (1999) and while we were writing the third (2003) without explanation, he was dismissed from this very prestigious and highly rewarding job. Likewise, another highly placed FIFA official – its director of marketing – who we duped into telling us more than he should have, was fired by FIFA President, Sepp Blatter, as after his re-election in 2002 he removed from his inner circle those he considered as enemies or at least those whose loyalty to the organisation (FIFA) was prioritised over their personal loyalty to him. While I have no proof that letting us in, facilitating our research and feeding us with insider knowledge was the sole reasons for their dismissals, I am nonetheless convinced that they were important contributory factors.

That FIFA and President Blatter wanted to take retribution on my co-author and I for the ensuing expose, I have absolutely no doubt as I still have a large bundle of legal papers served by them in a court in Switzerland in May 2003 in an attempt both to stop the publication of the third book in the trilogy, *Badfellas*, and suing us for liable. In the end, this attempt at legalistic bullying came to nothing, but at the time it was quite daunting to be facing the prospect of having to take on a hugely wealthy multinational organisation. While space in this chapter does not permit fuller consideration of the legal dimensions to investigative research, it is an area that should never be overlooked when planning and carrying out such work.

Corporate retribution can be hard and expensive, but the justice of the underworld can be even rougher. After the publication of *Scum Airways* (2002), my main gatekeeper received death threats from small-time mobsters and hardened football hooligans who were infuriated because he let me into and chaperoned me through their world. He had been given a pseudonym in the book, but the *cognoscenti* – the so-called Salford Mafia – recognised him through the detailed character description that I had given him. As alluded to earlier, the risk to him was compounded by the fact that the book had been written for a popular market and not as a relatively inaccessible academic thesis. At one stage, it seemed like half of Manchester were out to get 'Big Tommy'. Not long after the book was published enraged he telephoned me with the chilling message that because of me there was 'a bullet in Manchester' with his name on it. The situation only calmed down when his main tormentor was imprisoned for four years for football-related violence.[4] While both of these cases are regrettable, in my judgement each project was justifiable, both sociologically and most importantly in terms of the public interest.

The risk to research subjects has to be set against the chances that researchers themselves take when undertaking investigative fieldwork. The BSA warns that 'social researchers face a range of potential risks to their safety. Safety issues need to be considered in the design and conduct of social research projects and procedures should be adopted to reduce the risk to researchers' (2002, p. 3). Compared to the kinds of endeavours discussed in this chapter, the methods and mode of much contemporary sociology – sending out surveys, penning great thoughts or recycling the great thoughts of others from the sanctity of a university library, reinterpreting existing texts and related media analyses – are relatively risk-free occupations. Alone, such hands-off approaches cannot give us full access to and understanding of the complex worlds in which we live. If we are to follow Giddens (1976) wisdom (albeit metered out from his armchair), researchers must 'immerse' themselves and live the experience where structure and agency collide. By definition, this is far more risky than sitting in the library and, as I have argued elsewhere, ethnography is inherently perilous (Sugden, 1996). The risks multiply when the (under) worlds that you set out to access and share are at the margins of society and those that you research have something to hide. For instance, while doing boxing-related fieldwork in Northern Ireland during the 'troubles', I have been threatened by Irish Republican Army (IRA) gunmen. On several occasions during my time working with 'Big Tommy' and his gang during the 'Scum Airways' project, I have been threatened with extreme violence: not to mention the legalistic posturing of FIFA.

However, the level of risk can be minimised. The most important thing is for the researcher to be acutely aware that once in the field he or she is always at risk. In order to maximise understanding, fieldworkers should be ever alert to what is going on around them. To achieve this, they need to develop a highly tuned 'sociological antenna': using and extending our natural abilities to be acutely aware of what is going on at the centre, periphery and every corner of the social milieu that we find ourselves in. This is required for the generation of data, but it is also essential for self-preservation. For the purpose of generating open and fluid lines of communication, work hard to engender trust, but trust nobody. In the field, you are required to make decisions about who to be up-front with about your role and who not to tell, what is safe to do and who it is safe to be with. You need to make judgements on when it is safe to stay and when it is the time to leave and for this you also need an escape route.

One of the main reasons why I do not favour fully covert research – that is entering the field and posing as somebody else for all subjects, including gatekeepers – is that it offers no protection. There may come a time when the researcher may need to invoke the protection of his or her researchers' identity through a well-placed insider. Once you have let key gatekeepers know that you are doing research, this can act as an amnesty – a kind of 'get out of jail free' card – later in the investigation should you find yourself compromised. For instance, while studying football's black economy, on different occasions, I was accused of being under cover police, invited to take part in a variety of illegal scams and threatened with arrest as 'one of them'. At such times, it was valuable for me to reaffirm my researcher's role with my gatekeeper and make for the exit.

CONCLUSIONS

Getting under the surface soil of social life, digging deeply into and making coherent sense of the social experience of others, and translating those findings and interpretations into a universal language for widespread consumption are hugely challenging tasks. Taking account of the checks and balances outlined in this chapter, to help us meet these challenges I believe we do have much to learn from the traditions and techniques of investigative journalism. Kiernan's view of investigative journalism, that 'getting one's hands dirty is something that comes with the territory' (2000, p. 158) should not discourage sociologists from using similar approaches. Yes, it may mean occasionally getting our hands dirty, but so long as the grime is only skin deep, the product is clean and, above all, the story is in the public interest in the first place, it is usually worth the dig. What we need to do now is to debate and develop an ethical framework that guides us through rather than inhibits this important style of fieldwork. I offer this chapter as the beginning of this debate.

FIVE KEY READINGS

1. Kiernan, M. (2000). The regulatory and ethical framework. In H. De Burgh, (Ed.) *Investigative journalism. Context and practice* **(pp. 156–176). London: Routledge.**
For those primarily interested in investigative journalism, De Burgh's whole book is valuable. Kiernan's work is of particular relevance to the ethical debates featured in this chapter.

2. Mills, C. W. (1970). *The sociological imagination.* **Harmondsworth, UK: Pelican.**
This timeless classic should be compulsory reading on all sociology syllabuses. It is well worth reading, cover to cover, but of particular interest for this chapter is the final chapter on 'intellectual craftsmanship'.

3. Douglas, J. (1976). *Investigative social research: Individual and team field research.* **Beverly Hills, CA: Sage.**
The original and yet-to-be bettered text on investigative sociology that both provides a rationale for this approach and outlines its key features.

4. McDonald, I. (2002). Critical social research and political intervention: Moralistic versus radical approaches. In J. Sugden & A. Tomlinson (Eds.), *Power games. A critical sociology of sport.* **London: Routledge: 100–116.**
McDonald's chapter is particularly useful because it draws a distinction between research-informed practice that is geared towards enhancing the position of a particular moral/activist position and one in which the critical interpretation of dispassionately gathered evidence is informed by a radical and critical theoretical framework but not led by it.

5. Ward, S. (1997). Being objective about objectivity: The ironies of standpoint epistemological critiques of science. *Sociology 31*(4), 773–91.
For those who want to delve further into some of the more complex ontological and epistemological arguments summarised in this chapter, Ward's paper is essential reading.

NOTES

1. Some of the material in this chapter builds upon work with Alan Tomlinson previously published by us in *Power Games: A Critical Sociology of Sport* (2002) and a chapter of my own (Sugden, 2005) that appeared in a collection of essays on sport and ethics edited by Mike McNamee (2005).
2. For a fuller debate concerning this issue, See Ward (1997).
3. For examples of their brands of web-based investigative sport journalism, see Andrew Jennings' and Dave Zirin's websites, http://www.transparencyinsport.org/ and http://www.edgeofsports.com/
4. This character was released from prison on license in 2004 during which time he got into a fracas in a Salford public house and was shot and seriously injured. Incidentally he had also threatened violence against me during a fieldwork episode in Bangkok, Thailand, in 2002.

REFERENCES

BSA. (2002). *Statement of ethical practice*, British Sociological Association. Retrieved from http://www.britsoc.org.uk/about/ethic.htm. Accessed on 3rd September 2005.
Clegg, S. (2000). Theories of power. *Theory, Culture and Society, 17*(6), 139–147.

De Burgh, H. (2000). *Investigative journalism: Context and practice.* London: Routledge.

Douglas, J. (1976). *Investigative social research: Individual and team field research.* Beverly Hills, CA: Sage.

Gaber, I. (2003). Taming the daily beast. *Network*, 84, February 2–3.

Giddens, A. (1976). *New rules of sociological method.* London: Hutchinson.

Hesse, H. (1970). *The glass bead game.* London: Jonathan Cape.

Kaplan, J. (1975). *Lincoln Steffens: A biography.* London: Jonathan Cape.

Kiernan, M. (2000). The regulatory and ethical framework. In H. De Burgh (Ed.), *Investigative journalism. Context and practice* (pp. 156–176). London: Routledge.

Klein, A. (1993). *Little big men: Bodybuilding subculture and gender construction.* Albany, NY: State University of New York Press.

Lash, S. (1999). *Another modernity: A different rationality.* Oxford: Blackwell.

McDonald, I. (2002). Critical social research and political intervention: Moralistic versus radical approaches. In J. Sugden & A. Tomlinson (Eds.), *Power games. A critical sociology of sport* (pp. 100–116). London: Routledge.

McNamee, M. (2005). *Philosophy and the sciences of exercise, health and sport.* London: Routledge.

Mills, C. W. (1970). *The sociological imagination.* Harmondsworth, UK: Pelican.

Orwell, G. (Ed). (1994). Politics and the English Language. In *The penguin essays of George Orwell* (pp. 348–359). London: Penguin.

Pilger, J. (1999). *Hidden agendas.* London: Vantage.

Said, E. (1993). *Culture and imperialism.* London: Chatto and Windus.

Sugden, J. (1996). *Boxing and society. An international analysis.* Manchester: Manchester University Press.

Sugden, J. (2002). *Scum airways: Inside football's underground economy.* London: Mainstream.

Sugden, J. (2005). Is investigative sociology just investigative journalism? In M. McNamee (Ed.), *Philosophy and the sciences of exercise, health and sport.* London: Routledge.

Sugden, J., & Tomlinson, A. (1998). *FIFA and the contest for world football. Who rules the peoples' game?* London: Polity.

Sugden, J., & Tomlinson, A. (1999). *Great balls of fire. How big money is hi-jacking world football.* London: Mainstream.

Sugden, J., & Tomlinson, A. (2002). Critical sociology of sport: Theory and method. In J. Sugden & A. Tomlinson (Eds.), *Power games: A critical sociology of sport* (pp. 3–21). London: Routledge.

Sugden, J., & Tomlinson, A. (2003). *Badfellas. FIFA family at war.* London: Mainstream.

Tomlinson, A. (1997). Flattery and betrayal: Observations on qualitative and oral sources. In A. Tomlison & S. Flemming (Eds.), *Ethics, sport and leisure* (pp. 223–244). Aachen, Germany: Meyer and Meyer.

Wacquant, L. (1993). Positivism. In W. Outhwaite & T. Bottomore (Eds.), *The Blackwell dictionary of twentieth century social thought.* Oxford, UK: Blackwell.

Ward, S. (1997). Being objective about objectivity: The ironies of standpoint epistemological critiques of science. *Sociology*, *31*(4), 773–791.

Willis, P. (1977). *Learning to labour. How working class kids get working class jobs.* Farnborough, UK: Saxon House.

Woodwar, B., & Bernstein, C. (1981). *All the President's men.* London: Hodder and Stoughton.